KETO
MEAL PREP

31 DAYS MEAL PLAN

**THE COMPLETE KETO MEAL PREP GUIDE FOR BEGINNERS.
DELICIOUS AND EASY KETOGENIC RECIPES.**

RYAN CARTER

Table of Contents

INTRODUCTION

In a world where weight loss has been becoming a trend to many people and leading a healthy lifestyle a priority, there are so many fad diets promising effective weight loss have emerged such as the Atkins, Paleo, South Beach, and yes, the Ketogenic diet.

The philosophy of the keto diet revolves around ketone bodies as a main source of fuel. These ketones are produced by the liver from stored fats. Burning fats mean losing excess pounds, and that's good, but what is more surprising is getting the liver produce more ketones. For this to become possible, you need to follow a low carb diet, from 20-50 grams a day. This diet also requires high consumption of fat of at least 165 grams per day.

Protein also plays a part in the keto diet that requires at least 75 grams per day. Note though that the accurate ratio would depend on every person's particular needs.

The ketogenic diet also teaches a dieter mindful eating since it would involve growing awareness of making the right food choices. Mindful eating also teach you to eat healthy food make wise decisions if you want to keep the keto diet long term.

Now, you might be asking, do calories really matter in the keto diet? As most advocates would claim, calorie counting is really not an issue in this diet. But, if your goal is to lose weight, you still need to be aware of the amount of calories you take in a day. This is because even if you eat keto-friendly meals, but still ends up eating too much, you're still storing fats and you won't really lose weight. Keep in mind, the quality of calories consumed still play a major role in the keto diet. Succinct to say, calories matter on this diet. Even though you'll certainly feel less hungry and eat less, insufficient calories is still considered a piece of the puzzle in weight loss.

There are loads of weight loss myths, but given the keto diet, you will be sure that you're doing your weight and overall health a big favor. Not only does this diet helps in losing those unwanted pounds and stored fats, but it also gives you many health benefits that no other diet fads can give. So for now, give this diet a chance and see how your body and life transform.

CHAPTER 1 MEAL PREP AND KETO DIET

With proper meal planning, the ketogenic diet will help you lose more pounds and fats in no time at all. A lot of people have claimed to have lost weight because of this diet. This low-carb, high-fat diet helps effectively burn fat. It can also help in reversing type 2 diabetes and in losing excess body fat sans the usual cravings and hunger.

If you want to improve your health and achieve the body that you want, creating a meal plan with all keto-friendly food in it will be an ideal start towards your keto journey.

The ketogenic diet allows the body to produce "ketones". These are small fuel molecules that are produced when the body only consumes fewer amount of carbs. These ketones serve as a source of fuel for the body and brain. When on the keto diet, the body changes the fuel supply to mostly fat, thereby making your body a fat burning machine 24/7. This becomes way easier for fat stored to get burned. The moment the body produces ketones, you are entering a state called ketosis.

By lowering carb intake, the body is induced into a ketosis state. A properly-maintained and well-planned keto diet compels the body into ketosis, and this can be done through eating low carb food.

While the concept of consuming a low-carb and high fat diet may be easy, you can't just eat anything considered low-carb. You just don't reach out for that slab of bacon and eat it all day. A varied diet is still advised if you want to succeed in the Ketogenic Diet. Generally, you may consume food including fats and oils, vegetables, protein, seeds and nuts, dairy, and keto-friendly beverages.

Meal prepping is considered key to many successful diets. It is simply the process of preparing meals ahead of time. Doing so helps you save time thinking of what to eat, saves money, and helps you make healthy food choices. Many are intimidated by this food preparation process because they feel as if it's tedious. But once you do it, you will realize that it's easy after all.

The Benefits of Meal Prepping

Meal preparation involves different cooking techniques such as pan frying, roasting, boiling, slow cooking, glazing, deep frying, curing, and many other cooking techniques. This is no longer a new concept. Meal prepping is becoming more and more popular because of its many benefits:

1. You eat less

Too much carbohydrates is bad for you. In general, the body converts carbohydrates into energy, but consuming too much can increase your blood sugar level. This could lead to weight gain, slow metabolism, and even pave the way to different kinds of diseases. Meal prep helps you lose weight by controlling your food portions and limiting food that are not healthy.

2. You save a lot of money

An average fast food meal costs around $12. Eating 3 times a day in a fast food would yield to a whopping $36 a day. You multiply that for 30 days and you get to spend $1080 each month. Planning your meals in advance lets you buy supplies in bulk and lets you make a detailed list of food and ingredients to prepare. This eliminates frequent trips to the grocery store and do it just once or twice a week. You can save up to 50% on your grocery bill if you shop wisely and strategically by keeping yourself updated with sales and compare prices with different stores to get the most value for your money.

3. You'll feel encouraged to eat healthy at all times

It's difficult to eat healthy when you are at work. Meal prepping lets you enjoy good and nutrient dense food anytime, anywhere. When you prepare your food, you can just place them in containers and heat when ready to eat.

4. You don't have to waste food

You do not have to throw away your leftover beef or turkey. Meal prep allows you to transform leftover food into a whole new meal. You can use your leftover turkey for your wheat pasta or you can add it to your vegetable salad.

Meal Prepping Equipment and Food Storage

To ensure effective meal prepping, you should invest in the following items:

1. Mason jars, Bento boxes, and other food containers with air-tight lids meant for both liquid and solid food. You can use these to pre-cut ingredients until ready to use. For instance: mason jars can be used to store smoothies, shakes, and fruit juices in the fridge. Bento boxes, on the other hand, can be used to store dry ingredients such as cheese, rice, chopped onions, and hams among others.

2. Microwavable-safe and freezer containers. You should also invest in this one because they will come in handy when making soups and stews, or when precooking meals of large volume. All you have to do is cook meals beforehand, allow to cool, and then place in containers. Place in the fridge or freezer. Thaw and reheat as needed.

3. Baking trays, muffin tins cake racks, and other baking tools such as aluminum foil, parchment paper, saran wrap, muffin liners, and silicon baking mats among others. These will make pre-cooking and portioning easier.

4. Braising meat in the oven is a sound option if you're not going to use a pressure cooker or slow cooker. This is

beneficial when making large volumes of food good for the whole week. Invest in oven-safe cookware such as muffin tins, silicon baking sheet, cookie tray, and deep baking dishes.

5. Stickers, dry erase markers, sticky notes, papers, sharpies, and transparent adhesive tape. These will help in labeling containers when meal prepping. When you label them using these labeling implements, you must add details such as the date dishes are made and until when they're best consumed, ingredients used, portions, etc. Properly labeling ensures that all your prepared meals will not go unused.

6. Colanders and strainers. These are mainly used for draining and rinsing ingredients. These tools are helpful when draining pasta and rinsing vegetables and rice. Pro tip: buy different sizes for different purposes. Metal strainers are perfect when draining fried food, while plastic colanders are for rinsing fresh produce.

7. Non-stick pans, pots, and griller. These are perfect if you want your food with lesser amount of oil. The best thing about these pans is that you can fry fish even without the use of oil. Best part is they won't stick to the pan.

8. Blender and food processor. This can be a stovetop or an immersion. These will help chopping ingredients hassle free. Remember, meal prepping entails chopping, slicing, grinding, and mincing ingredients. Using these appliances will lessen the stress when preparing dishes in large quantities.

9. Oven-proof skillets – these skillets are perfect for baking and frying. You can also use these to brown meats and then bake them.

10. Mixing Bowls – there are three types that you will need – small, medium, and large. These are ideal for mixing sauces, ingredients, and other food that would require the use of different bowl sizes.

Money Saving Tips in Meal Prepping

1. Prepare a meal plan every week.

Doing this will help you stick to your keto diet and ultimately reach your goals. The first thing you need to do is to list all keto-friendly ingredients and how much calories you intend to follow. Your daily calorie needs would depend on factors, such as weight, age, height, gender, and exercise level.

The moment you determine your daily caloric needs, know how much weight you want to lose. In order to lose 1 pound in a week, you would have to get rid of at least 500 calories from your daily intake. To lose 2 pounds a week, you need to consume 1000 calories less than your daily calorie needs. Take for instance, if you need 2500 calories in a day, consume 1500 calories to lose 2 pounds a week or you can consume 2000 calories and burn the remaining 500 calories through physical activity.

Afterwards, it is time to start planning your meals. Write your meal plan and stick it where you can easily see it. There are also different meal prepping apps that you can use such as Yummly, Pinterest, Pepperplate, Google Calendar, Food Print, and Menu Planner.

2. Create a weekly grocery list

This habit will help you save time and money. After creating your weekly meal plan, list down all ingredients needed for the recipes for a week. You can either write these in a notebook or use apps such as AnyList, Shopping List, Ziplist, Grocery IQ, Epicurous,Flipp, Out of Milk, Cozi Family Organizer, Trello, and Buy Me A Pie among others.

3. Chop the vegetables in advance

In meal prepping, it is vital that all ingredients are chopped and stored in zip-lock bags for easier cooking. Here's a list of vegetables that you can chop days before cooking them and their best storage time:

- Onions – best kept for up to 7 days

- Cauliflower – best kept for up to 7 days
- Broccoli – best kept for up to 5 to 7 days
- Cucumber – best kept for up to 2 days
- Cabbage – best kept for up to 7 days
- Mushroom – best kept for up to 2 days
- Lettuce – best kept for up to 10 days
- Asparagus – best kept for up to 3 to 5 days
- Eggplant – best kept for up to 12 days
- Tomatoes – best kept for up to 2 days
- Kale – best kept for up to 7 days
- Carrots – best kept for up to 14 days
- Baby Spinach – best kept for up to 3 days
- Celery – best kept for up to 14 days

4. Make sure to label everything.

This is so you can avoid food and ingredient mix up. Place the name of the recipe and the date on the labels. If prepping the ingredients ahead of time, you may attach the recipe on the container or name the dish that you will use those ingredients for.

5. Pick a day to cook all meals for the week on that day.

This may seem overwhelming, but it gets easier over time. You can chop all the ingredients of all your meals in, say, 30 to 40 minutes. This will save you time as it usually take you 10 minutes to chop the ingredients of just one meal. If you want to save more time, you can purchase a food processor.

4. Place salads in a mason jar.

This will prevent the salad from sogging and is a time saver, too. You can simply layer the vegetables in each jar.

5. Use different sauces for the same meal

Eating the same meal week after week can make you feel bored and make you want to quit meal prep altogether. To avoid this, it's best to use different sauces for the same meals. For example, you can cook shrimps with garlic sauce this week and then use a sweet and sour sauce next week.

6. Bake "hard-boiled" eggs

To save time, you can bake your "hard-boiled" eggs. Simply place a dozen or two dozen eggs in a muffin tin. Bake in the oven at 350F for 30 minutes. Then, place the eggs in cold water for 5 to 10 minutes before you peel them.

7. Check your produce regularly.

Make sure to monitor the status of your produce every day so you'd prevent them from going stale.

8. Take note of the dishes that you like and those that you don't.

Make it a habit to take note of the recipes that you actually like. This way, you get to prepare these dishes often. Also, take note of the meal prep methods that work well for you.

Lastly, have fun meal prepping. It would be a bit tedious in the beginning, but you can surely get the hang of it.

KETO ON A BUDGET

Being and eating healthy should never be a threat to your wallet. Eating healthy only means that you have to be smart especially when buying food. Here is a list of tried and tested saving techniques to buying Keto:

1. Bulk Up.

   - When grocery shopping, it is always a good idea to buy in bulk. In Keto, you will always need eggs, bacon, and chicken breasts. So buy a lot of these and store up.

2. Make your own.

   - It's time to ditch those store bought salad dressings and nut butter. Making your own will not only help you manage your carbohydrates, it will also save you a lot of money. Invest in a food processor and spiralizer to help you make your own nut butters and vegetable pasta.

3. Freeze.

   - When preparing Keto meals, always save up your excess and refrigerate them. Doing this will ensure that no food goes to waste and that you will always have something ready to heat and eat on the fridge. Always remember to mark dates on your frozen food.

4. Go fatty.

   - Fattier meat cuts are least expensive compared to leaner, red cuts. And in Keto diet, this is heaven. You will not only meet your fat requirement, you'll also be saving money on your meats.

5. Opt for a healthier drink – Water.

   - Skip the diet soda or any soda. Just drink natural, drinking water. Go for teas and coffees, too. Spike your teas and coffees with some olive oil or ghee to make them Keto friendly. You could also experiment by adding different flavors on your teas and coffees.

6. Buy frozen.

   - When buying vegetables, always choose frozen ones. Frozen vegetables usually last longer than fresh ones. They are also relatively cheaper than fresh ones. Zucchini, spinach, and lettuce are your go-to greens in the Keto diet. So always keep them handy.

7. Prepare a meal plan.

   - Preparing a meal plan will save you lots of time in grocery shopping and meal preparation. It will also ensure that you are on track on your Keto diet.

8. Coupons.

   - There's nothing wrong with scouring the newspapers for coupons. And with the rise of technology, coupons are also available online. Collect coupons and use them to pay for what shopped.

9. Look for deals and sales.

   - When shopping, always look for deals, sales, and discounts. This can help you buy more than your money's worth. Look what vegetables are in season and buy them in bulk.

10. Go online.

   - Join Keto themed groups online and sign up for online markets. A community of Keto dieters can help you find the best deals when it comes to specialty ingredients. You can also share recipes and discuss about the best alternative to a pricey ingredient.

The Keto Grocery List

In Keto, there are few things that you should always stock. Keeping these items on hand will help you turn any dish into a Keto dish. Prices added are dollar/pound. Based on

Basic Keto Necessities

- Eggs about 68 cents per dozen
- Bacon (4.8 USD)
- Chicken (whole – 1.3USD; breasts – 3.3USD; 1.5USD)
- Almonds (12-15USD/kilo)
- Broccoli (1.6USD)
- Spinach (2.56-4.99 USD/ 6oz package)
- Lettuce (1.79USD/package)
- Butter (Salted – 3.7USD)

If you want a more advanced Keto dining experience, stock up on these items too:

- Tuna (fillet – 18.99USD/lb.)
- Ground Beef – (2.8USD)
- Sardines (12-14USD/carton)
- Salmon (fillets – 11.99USD/lb.)
- Pork rinds
- Pork shoulders
- Cheese (Cheddar – 5.6USD)
- Ham
- Sour cream

- Greek yogurt (2.5USD/ 32oz.)
- Avocado (1.2USD per piece)
- Cumin (4.4-4.6USD/kilo)
- Cauliflower (1.49-2.79USD/lbs.)
- Asparagus (3.99USD/lb.)
- Mushrooms (1.5USD/ 8.oz)
- Blueberries (2.7USD per package)
- Walnuts
- Cayenne
- Coconut oil
- Olive oil
- Basil
- Garlic powder
- Beef tenderloin (2.99USD/lb.)
- Cilantro (0.99USD per bunch)

Specialty Ingredients:

- Stevia
- Erythiol
- Xanthum gum
- Chia seeds

CHAPTER 2 BREAKFAST RECIPES

Recipe #1 - Baked Eggs Wrapped in Bacon

Ingredients:

- 12 pieces long streaky bacon, torn to fit into individual cups of two 1¾" x ¾" muffin tins
- 12 pieces small or tiny fresh eggs at room temperature
- Salt and pepper to taste

Directions:

1. Preheat oven to 190°C or 375°F for at least 10 minutes.
2. Line each muffin cup with streaky bacon, covering bottoms and sides well.
3. Crack eggs directly into each muffin cup. Season lightly with salt and pepper.
4. Bake for 20 minutes or until bacon crisps and yolks are set.
5. Remove muffin tins immediately from the oven. Set on wire rack to cool for 5 minutes, loosely tented with aluminum foil.
6. Carefully extract bacon and eggs from muffin tins. Serve two pieces per person.
7. To reheat: place a sealed bag (one portion) into microwave oven. Set at highest heat setting for 3 to 5seconds only. Remove eggs and bacon from bags before serving.

Recipe #2 – Avocado, Broccoli, and Bacon in a Pan

Ingredients:

- 3 rashers of bacon

- 1 cup of broccoli florets

- 4 pieces asparagus stems

- 1 piece avocado, sliced thinly

- 2 eggs

- Rock salt

- Ground pepper

Directions:

1. Cook bacon in a frying pan on medium low until it grease.

2. Place the avocado slices in the same pan and cook in bacon fat until crisped. (About 2 minutes per side)

3. Remove the bacon and the avocado slices and then cook the eggs. Season eggs with salt and pepper.

4. When eggs are almost cooked, add the broccoli florets and the asparagus into the pan. Cover and cook for 3 minutes.

5. Plate the eggs and vegetable with a side of bacon and avocado fries.

Recipe #3 – Avocado Breakfast Toast

Ingredients:

- 1 tablespoon unsalted butter

- a slice of bread, pre toasted

- Ripe avocado, peeled, halved, seeded, and thinly sliced

- A drizzle of olive oil

- Sesame seeds

- Crushed red pepper flakes, for garnish and optional

- Kosher salt and ground black pepper, to taste

Directions:

1. Spread some unsalted butter on the toast.

2. Place thinly sliced avocado on top.

3. Dress with some olive oil and top with red pepper flakes and sesame seeds.

4. Season with salt and pepper.

Recipe #4 - Spicy and Cheesy Sausage

Ingredients:

- 12 oz frozen hot pork sausage, thawed

- 2 garlic cloves, finely chopped

- 1/3 cup onion, chopped

- 1 cup red bell pepper, chopped

- 1/4 teaspoon salt

- 1 1/2 cups Mexican cheese blend, shredded

- 1 1/2 cups all-purpose flour

- 1/4 teaspoon red pepper flakes, crushed

- 3 eggs

- 1 cup milk

Directions:

1. Heat oven to a temperature of 425°F. Use cooking spray or shortening to grease the bottom and sides of a 3-quart glass baking dish measuring 13x9-inches with shortening or cooking spray.

2. In a 12-inch skillet, cook the sausage, garlic, and onion over medium heat while frequently stirring until the meat no longer shows traces of pink. Drain and then stir in the bell pepper.

3. Remove skillet from heat. Using a wire whisk, beat flour, crushed red pepper, salt, eggs and milk in large bowl until consistency is smooth. Pour mixture into the baking dish and then spoon the sausage mixture over the batter. Finally, sprinkle with cheese.

4. Bake until top the top turns golden brown, which should take 22 to 27 minutes. This makes 12 servings.

Recipe #5 – Buttered Omelet

Ingredients:

- 3 eggs, soaked in hot water for 5 minutes
- 1/2 tsp. fresh chives, chopped
- 1 1/2 tsps. butter, set at room temperature
- Salt

Directions:

1. Crack eggs into a bowl. Season with salt and beat with a fork or a beater.

2. Heat a non-stick skillet over medium heat. Melt around a teaspoon of butter and brush it around the pan.

3. Pour eggs into the pan and stir with spatula for several seconds. When eggs starting to form some solid parts, lift the pan and move it slightly to spread raw eggs to the other parts of the pan. Nudge parts of spatula to form round omelet. Let it sit for 10 seconds without stirring.

4. Shake the pan to loosen the egg. Get your spatula and fold a third part of the omelet. Transfer it to a plate and fold again to create a triple-folded omelet. Coat with the half-teaspoon butter and top with chives. Serve hot.

Recipe #6 - Breakfast Sausage

Ingredients

- 2 teaspoons dried sage

- 2 pounds of ground pork

- 1/4 teaspoon dried marjoram

- 1/8 teaspoon crushed red pepper flakes

- 1 tablespoon brown sugar

- 1 pinch ground cloves

- 2 teaspoons salt

- 1 teaspoon ground black pepper

Directions:

1. Combine all ingredients except the ground pork in a small bowl. Mix well.

2. In a large bowl, place the ground pork and then add in the mixed spices. Thoroughly mix using your hands and then form into patties.

3. In a large skillet, sauté the patties over moderate to high heat for about 5 minutes for each side, or until the internal temperature of the pork reaches 160 degrees F.

Recipe #7 - Keto Breakfast

Ingredients:

- 3 eggs

- 2 bacon rashers

- 2 tbsp of sour cream

- 1 tbsp of butter

- 1/8 tsp of black pepper

- 1/8 tsp of paprika

- ¼ tsp of salt

Directions:

1. Crack eggs into a pan and butter. Cook eggs on medium-high heat while stirring constantly.

2. Alternately stir the eggs on and off the heat with a 30 seconds interval. When the eggs are nearly done, remove pan from heat.

3. Once you removed the eggs from the heat, immediately add a tablespoon of sour cream into the eggs and season with salt, paprika and pepper.

4. On another pan, fry the bacon rashers until golden brown.

5. Place eggs and bacon on a plate and garnish eggs.

Recipe #8 - Egg and Cheese

Ingredients:

- 5 large eggs
- 2 cups sliced cheddar cheese

Directions:

1. Heat the oven to 350F. Place in a muffin tray.

2. Bake for 10 minutes.

3. Let the eggs cool for a few minutes. Remove the egg shells and slice each egg into three. Place each egg in a ziplock bag.

4. Divide the cheddar cheese among the five ziplock bags.

5. Store in the refrigerator up to five days. You may or may not heat the eggs before serving.

Recipe #9 - Breakfast Jerk Chicken

Ingredients:

- 5 pieces of chicken breasts
- ¼ cup of chopped cilantro
- 1/4 cup of Jamaican seasoning
- Cooking spray
- Pinch of salt
- Pinch of pepper

Directions:

1. Coat each chicken breast with Jamaican seasoning. Season with salt and pepper.
2. Grease a skillet with a cooking spray. Add the chicken and cook for five to seven minutes.
3. Add cilantro and cook for another 10 minutes.
4. Remove the skillet from heat and let it cool for a while.
5. Divide the chicken among seven microwaveable containers. Store the containers in the refrigerator up to five days. Heat each container in a microwave oven before serving.

Recipe #10 - Baked Ham and Cheese Omelet

Ingredients:

- 1 cup ham or deli ham, cooked, chopped
- 6 eggs
- 1/2 cup all-purpose flour
- 1 cup sharp cheddar cheese, shredded
- 1 cup milk
- Salt and pepper

Directions

1. Preheat oven to 450 degrees F.
2. Combine eggs and milk. Beat until fluffy.
3. Add flour and season with pepper and salt. Beat until well-blended.
4. Grease a 13x9-inch oven dish with butter. Pour eggs into the oven dish.
5. Bake for 15 minutes until set. Be careful because some ovens can cook eggs within 6 minutes.
6. Top with chopped ham or arrange ham slices evenly on the egg. Top with cheese.
7. Bake for additional 5 minutes until cheese melts.
8. Transfer to a serving dish. Cut into pieces and serve.

Recipe #11 - Herbed Mushrooms and Eggs

Ingredients:

- 3 Tbsp. olive oil
- 6 large eggs
- 24 large button mushrooms, trimmed and chopped
- 2/3 cup chopped red onion
- 2 small garlic cloves, minced
- 1 ½ tsp dried thyme
- ¾ tsp dried oregano
- ½ cup crumbled feta cheese
- Sea salt
- Freshly ground black pepper

Directions:

1. Place a cast-iron skillet over high flame and heat through. Add 1 ½ tablespoons olive oil and sauté the onion and garlic until tender.

2. Stir in the mushrooms and herbs then sauté until mushrooms are fork tender. Transfer to a platter.

3. Wipe the skillet and heat the remaining olive oil. Break the eggs into the skillet and cook two at a time, sunny-side up. Season lightly with salt and pepper. Once almost set, sprinkle in ¼ cup feta cheese.

4. Cover the skillet and cook for 30 seconds or until the cheese melts. Transfer the eggs onto the mushrooms and add the remaining cheese.

Recipe #12 - Basil Scrambled Eggs

Ingredients:

- 3 tsp olive oil

- 6 large eggs

- 3 Tbsp. julienned fresh basil

Directions:

1. Whisk the eggs and basil in a bowl until frothy. Set aside.

2. Place a cast-iron skillet over high flame and heat through. Add the olive oil and sauté the garlic until tender. Reduce to low flame.

3. Pour in the basil-egg mixture and scramble lightly until fluffy. Transfer to a plate.

Recipe #13 - Baked Omelet with Cheese

Ingredients

- 4 eggs

- 4 green onions, sliced

- 12 oz. cheese, sliced into half-inch cubes

- 1/4 cup water

- 1 bell pepper, diced

- 1 cup cooked ham, diced

- 2 tbsps. butter

- Salt

Directions:

1. Preheat oven to 400 degrees F.

2. Combine water and eggs. Season with salt.

3. Heat an ovenproof pan. Melt butter for sautéing.

4. Sauté onions, bell pepper, and ham for 3 minutes. Spread sautéed ingredients evenly on the pan.

5. Pour egg mixture over the sautéed ingredients. Top with cheese.

6. Bake for 20 minutes until cheese melts. Garnish with parsley if preferred before serving.

Recipe #14 - Cinnamon Pancakes

Ingredients:

- 3 Tbsp coconut flour

- 6 large eggs

- 2/3 tsp baking soda

- 1/3 tsp ground nutmeg

- 1 ½ tsp ground cinnamon

- ¾ cup coconut milk

- 1 ½ tsp freshly squeezed lemon juice

- 3 tsp raw honey

- 3 Tbsp coconut oil

Directions:

1. Sift the dry ingredients together into a large bowl. Set aside.

2. Beat the eggs, lemon juice, honey and coconut milk in another bowl, then gradually pour into the bowl of dry ingredients. Mix until thoroughly incorporated. Batter may be refrigerated.

3. Place a pancake griddle over medium flame and coat with some coconut oil. Ladle about a quarter cup of the batter onto the hot griddle and cook for 1 minute per side.

4. Transfer pancakes onto a platter and keep covered as you cook the remaining batter.

Recipe #15 - Ham and Egg Cups

Ingredients:

- 8 pieces quail eggs, fresh

- 4 slices sweet ham, sliced into wide slivers

- 1 slice, thick keto-friendly bread, quartered

- 2 tsp. cheddar cheese, grated

- white pepper, to taste

Directions:

1. Preheat oven to 350°F. Place 4 paper liners into large muffin tins. Set aside.

2. Place 1 bread quarter into base of each muffin cup. Break 2 quail eggs on top and sprinkle equal portions of cheese. Bake these for 10 to 15 minutes, or until eggs are set. Remove muffin tins from oven immediately.

3. Carefully remove each cup from muffin tins, and cool slightly for easier handling.

4. Season with pepper before serving. Serve warm.

Recipe #16 - Avocado and Egg Salad

Ingredients:

- 1 avocado, ripe, pitted, peeled
- 2 tablespoons of mayonnaise
- 1 egg, hard-boiled
- 1 teaspoon of garlic powder
- paprika
- 1/8 teaspoon of lemon juice, fresh
- salt and pepper
- fresh parsley

Directions:

1. Cut avocado into chunks.
2. Chop hard-boiled egg and then add to avocado. Add remaining ingredients.
3. Let stand or refrigerate, but not for very long – an hour will do.
4. Serve on a bed of lettuce and then sprinkle some paprika on top.

Recipe #17 – Spicy Omelet

Ingredients:

- 3/4 cup red onion, minced finely

- 2 tbsps. fresh cilantro leaves, minced

- 2 tbsps. canola oil

- 1 Serrano chile, seeded if you don't prefer spicy, minced

- 6 eggs

- 3/4 tsp. each of paprika and turmeric

- Kosher salt and black pepper

Directions:

1. Crack eggs into a bowl. Beat them for a minute until lathery.

2. Add and stir onions, turmeric, cilantro, paprika and chile. Mix well.

3. Season with a pinch of salt and freshly ground black pepper.

4. Heat oil in a 12-inch pan over medium heat.

5. Pour egg mixture in the pan. Mix with a spatula in circular motions, distributing the solid ingredients evenly into the pan. Cover and continue cooking for around 3 minutes.

6. Transfer cooked eggs into a 12-inch platter by letting it slide off the pan. Cooked side should be on the pan. Cover the plate with the pan. Flip them over so the uncooked side will land on the bottom of the plate. Cook for another minute without covering.

Recipe #18 - Breakfast Sausage Casserole

Ingredients:

- 1 pound of ground pork sausage

- 8 ounces of shredded mild Cheddar cheese

- 1/2 teaspoon salt

- 1 teaspoon of mustard powder

- 4 beaten eggs

- 6 slices of white bread, toasted and cubed

- 2 cups of milk

Directions:

1. Crumble pork sausage into a medium-sized skillet and then cook over medium heat settings until meat is evenly brown. Drain.

2. Grease a 9 x13 (inches) baking dish.

3. Combine mustard powder, eggs, milk, and salt in a medium bowl. Mix well and then add the bread cubes, cheese, and sausage. Stir to evenly coat. Pour mixture into baking dish and then cover. Chill in the fridge overnight or for about 8 hours.

4. Preheat oven to a temperature of 350 degrees F. Cover, and then bake for 45 minutes to an hour. Uncover, and then lower heat to 325 degrees F. Bake for 30 minutes more, or until casserole sets.

Recipe #19 - Creamy Scrambled Egg

Ingredients:

- Buttermilk

- Heavy cream

- Coconut Oil or Butter

- Eggs

Directions:

1. Add and combine a tablespoon of buttermilk to half a cup of heavy cream.

2. Leave cream loosely covered to ferment at room temperature for about 12 hours. Set aside

3. Crack eggs in a bowl and beat with fork.

4. Pre heat and grease a small pan.

5. Add a tablespoon of fermented heavy cream into the egg mixture. Fold until well combined.

6. Pour eggs into the pan and cook until done. Stir eggs constantly to avoid overcooking. Serve.

Recipe #20 - Avocado Lime Salad

Ingredients:

- 2 medium-size avocados, peeled, pitted and diced
- 1 medium-size green bell pepper, chopped
- 1 sweet onion, chopped
- 1 ripe tomato, chopped
- 1/2 cup of lime juice
- 1/4 cup of fresh cilantro, chopped
- salt and pepper

Directions:

1. Combine avocados, bell pepper, onion, tomato, lime juice, and cilantro in a medium bowl. Gently toss the mixture until coating is even.

2. Add salt and pepper to your liking.

Recipe #21 - Avocado-Tomato Salad

Ingredients:

- 2 avocados, ripe, diced
- 1/2 cup nicoise olives, chopped roughly
- 2 ripe beefsteak tomatoes, diced
- 1 cup of canned chickpeas, drained, rinsed and then drained again
- 1/4 cup champagne vinegar
- 2 tablespoons of flat-leaf parsley, roughly torn
- 1/4 cup extra-virgin olive oil
- 1/2 teaspoon of smoked paprika
- 1 teaspoon of ground cumin
- Salt
- black pepper, freshly ground
- 2 ounces of tortilla chips, blue corn variety

Directions:

1. In a large bowl, gently toss the avocados, olives, tomatoes, parsley, chickpeas, olive oil, vinegar, paprika, cumin, salt and pepper.

2. Crumble the tortilla chips over the salad and then serve. This makes 4 servings.

Recipe #22 - Egg White Omelet

Ingredients:

- One 32-oz. container refrigerated egg white substitute, pasteurized
- 2 tbsps. mushrooms, chopped
- 2 tbsps. onion, chopped
- 2 tbsps. green bell pepper, chopped
- Salt and black pepper
- Cooking spray

Directions:

1. Grease a 9x5-inch oven-safe loaf pan with cooking spray.
2. Place mushrooms, green bell pepper and onions in the pan, ensuring they are evenly distributed. Toss lightly to mix.
3. Eason with freshly ground black pepper and salt.
4. Pour eggs to the onion mixture.
5. Bake in a microwave for 3 minutes on high setting.
6. Remove the pan out of the oven and stir. Mix well with other ingredients.
7. Bring back to the microwave and cook for another 3 minutes.
8. In case some parts are still runny, slice the egg loaf in chunks then turnover. Cook for 30 minutes.
9. Season again with salt and pepper to adjust taste.

Recipe #23 - Asparagus and Prosciutto

Ingredients:

- 3 bunches of asparagus, woody ends trimmed
- 6 slices of prosciutto
- 2 tablespoons of olive oil
- 250 grams of finely chopped cherry tomato
- 1 tablespoon white wine vinegar
- A pinch of caster sugar
- 2 anchovy fillets, finely chopped, drained on paper towel
- More olive oil, for greasing asparagus
- 55gs (about a third of a cup) toasted pine nuts
- Salt and pepper, to taste

Directions:

1. Preheat oven to 400°F. Then, use non-stick baking paper to line baking tray. Place prosciuttos on the tray. Bake until crisp (around 5 minutes). Set aside to cool slightly (around for 5 minutes), and then use fingers to break prosciuttos into large pieces.

2. For the dressing, whisk tomato, anchovy, vinegar, olive oil and sugar together in a small bowl. Add salt and pepper to taste.

3. Preheat chargrill or barbecue grill on high settings. Brush asparagus with olive oil. Add salt and pepper to taste. Cook asparagus on grill, occasionally turning (usually after about two minutes), or until tender crisp and bright green.

4. To serve, divide asparagus among plates. Drizzle with the dressing and then top with crispy prosciuttos and pine nuts.

Recipe #24 - Grilled Asparagus

Ingredients:

- 1 lb fresh asparagus spears, ends trimmed
- 1 tablespoon of olive oil
- salt and pepper

Directions:

1. Preheat grill for high heat.

2. Coat the asparagus spears lightly with olive oil. You can use your hands to roll them over. Add salt and pepper to taste.

3. Grill over high heat for around 2 to 3 minutes, or to tenderness you prefer.

Recipe #25 - Pepper Mushroom Eggs

Ingredients:

- 3 large eggs
- 4 mushrooms
- Red bell peppers
- Spinach
- A few slices of ham
- Ghee or coconut oil
- Salt and pepper to taste

Directions:

1. Chop or dice the ham and the vegetables into smaller pieces.

2. Melt half a tablespoon of butter into a frying pan. Add the ham and vegetables and sauté.

3. Add the remaining butter on another frying pan. Fry the egg on the greased pan over medium heat. Stir eggs to avoid overcooking.

4. Season eggs with some salt and pepper.

5. Mix the sautéed vegetables and ham with the scrambled eggs and leave to cook. Serve.

Recipe #26 - Parmesan Buttered Asparagus

Ingredients:

- 3/4 cup Parmesan cheese, grated

- 1 tablespoon butter

- 1 lb fresh asparagus spears, ends trimmed

- 1/4 cup of olive oil

- salt and pepper

Directions:

1. Over medium heat settings, place olive oil in a large skillet and then melt butter. Add the asparagus spears.

2. Cook for about 10 minutes, or to desired firmness, stirring occasionally. Remove excess oil, and then sprinkle Parmesan cheese on top. Add salt and pepper to taste.

Recipe #27 - Romaine and Turkey Bacon Salad

Ingredients:

- 1 cup of diced ham

- 4 pieces of cherry tomatoes

- Some bleu cheese

- 2 large eggs, hardboiled

- Romaine lettuce, coarsely chopped

- Diced avocado

- 2 rashers of turkey bacon

For the salad dressing:

- A tablespoon of olive oil

- A tablespoon of organic apple cider vinegar

- A teaspoon of lemon juice

- A teaspoon of Dijon mustard

- A clove of garlic, crushed

- Salt and pepper to taste

Directions:

1. Combine salad ingredients in a bowl. Mix salad dressing ingredients in another bowl.

2. Plate the salad and drizzle some salad dressing on top. Toss salad to mix. Serve.

Recipe #28 - Cucumber Salad

Ingredients:

- 2 large cucumbers, sliced
- Salt and pepper
- 1 tablespoon apple cider vinegar
- 1 cup of honeydew, sliced

Directions:

1. Place all the ingredients in a large bowl. Mix well.
2. Then, divide the salad between two mason jars.
3. Close the mason jars. Store the mason jars in the refrigerator up to three days. You can eat this dish cold. You can simply put the mason jar in your lunch bag.

Recipe #29 - Broccoli Frittata

Ingredients:

- 5 cups of cooked broccoli
- 5 egg whites
- Garlic powder
- Salt, as needed
- 2 tablespoons of olive oil

Directions:

1. Beat the eggs in a bowl. Then, add the garlic powder and salt.
2. Heat the oil in a skillet over medium heat. Add the broccoli and cook for two to five minutes. Add a little bit of pepper and salt. Once the broccoli is tender, pour the egg mixture over.
3. Cook for three to five minutes, folding occasionally.
4. Remove from heat and let it cool for five to ten minutes.

Recipe #30 - Cauliflower Hash

Ingredients:

- 3 egg whites
- ½ teaspoon of garlic salt
- ½ cup of olive oil
- 1 head of shredded cauliflower
- 2 tablespoon of flour

Directions:

1. Place the shredded cauliflower for three minutes. Set aside.
2. Place the egg whites, garlic salt, cauliflower, and flour in a large bowl. Stir the mixture well. Then, form four patties out of the cauliflower mixture.
3. Heat the olive oil over medium heat. Add the patties to the pan and cook for four minutes each side.

Recipe #31 - Keto Vegan Salad

Ingredients:

- Cauliflower florets

- Finely diced parsley

- 3 sprigs of finely diced mint leaves

- Diced cherry tomatoes

- A slice of lemon, diced

- A tablespoon of olive oil

- Salt and pepper to taste

Directions:

1. Process the cauliflower heads in a food process. The texture should be couscous like.

2. In a bowl, mix together the processed cauliflower heads, the cherry tomatoes, the diced lemon, the diced parsley and mint leaves.

3. Dress salad with some olive oil.

4. Season with some salt and pepper.

CHAPTER 3 KETO LUNCH RECIPES

Recipe #32 - Beef Stroganoff with Mushrooms

Ingredients:

- 1 and 1/2 pounds of round steak, cubed and cut into thin strips
- Special seasoning mix
- All-purpose flour
- 8 ounces mushrooms, fresh, sliced
- 2 tablespoons of butter
- 2 tablespoons of olive oil
- 1 onion, medium, sliced
- 1 can beef broth
- 1 can of cream of mushroom soup
- Salt and black pepper to taste
- 1 cup of sour cream
- Egg noodles, cooked
- Special Seasoning blend:
- 1/4 cup of black pepper
- 1 cup salt
- 1/4 cup of garlic powder

Direction:

1. For the Stroganoff Sprinkle steak strips with this recipe's special seasoning blend to lightly cover them. Dust seasons meat strips with flour.

2. In a large pan, heat butter and olive oil, and then quickly brown strips of beef on both sides. Remove steak strips.

3. Add mushrooms and onion slices to the pan drippings and sauté for a couple of minutes until onion slices are tender. Then, sprinkle with a teaspoon of flour.

4. Place steak strips back into the pan containing the mushrooms and onion. Add beef broth and mushroom soup. Cover pan and then cook for around 30 minutes over low heat. Add salt and pepper. In the last few minutes before serving, stir in the sour cream. Serve stroganoff over cooked egg noodles. This makes 4 servings.

5. For the seasoning blend, mix all ingredients together thoroughly and then place inside an airtight container. This blend can be stored for up to 6 months.

Recipe #33 - Broccoli Soup

Ingredients:

- 4 cups chicken stock, low-salt
- 1 onion, large, chopped
- 1 1/2 lbs. fresh broccoli
- 1 carrot, chopped
- 4 tbsps. butter, sitting at room temperature
- 3 tbsps. all-purpose flour
- 1/2 cup cream
- Salt and black pepper

Directions:

1. Set a heavy pot on medium to high heat. Melt all the butter.

2. Sauté onion, broccoli and carrots. Season with freshly ground black pepper. Continue cooking for 6 minutes until onion is translucent.

3. Add flour and cook for a minute or until golden. Pour stock and stir. Bring to boil.

4. Remove cover and continue simmering for 15 minutes until broccoli is tender. Pour cream.

5. Puree the mixture by using an immersion blender. Season with pepper and salt. Cover again. Serve.

Recipe #34 - Chicken Strips and Broccoli

Ingredients:

- 1 lb. chicken breast, skinless and boneless, sliced into strips
- 1/2 cup chicken broth, low-salt
- 4 cups broccoli florets
- 2 tbsps. Dijon mustard
- 1 tbsp. soy sauce, light variant
- 1 tbsp. olive oil
- 1 garlic clove, minced

Directions:

1. Combine soy sauce and broth. Set aside.
2. Set pan over medium-high heat. Heat oil then sauté garlic and broccoli. Cook until crispy.
3. Remove cooked broccoli from the pan. Transfer to another plate, but keep warm.
4. Cook chicken on the same pan for 4 minutes until cooked through.
5. Pour broth and soy sauce mix. Mix well. Bring to boil.
6. Reduce heat to medium low setting. Add mustard. Mix well.
7. Put broccoli back to the mixture and mix.
8. Simmer while stirring constantly until completely cooked.

Recipe #35 - Cream of Asparagus Soup

Ingredients:

- 1 ½ lb asparagus, rinsed and trimmed

- 1 ½ cups whole milk

- 1 ½ cups water

- 3 Tbsp chopped fresh Italian parsley

- Sea salt

- Freshly ground black pepper

Directions:

1. Pour the water and milk into a saucepan and add the asparagus. Season with a pinch of salt and pepper, then mix well.

2. Place the saucepan over high flame and bring to a boil. Once boiling, reduce to medium low flame and let simmer.

3. Simmer the soup, uncovered for about 8 minutes or until the asparagus is fork tender.

4. Turn off the heat and allow to cool slightly. Then, transfer the asparagus to a food processor and add some of the liquid. Blend until smooth, then return to the saucepan and stir to combine.

5. Reheat until warmed through and season to taste with salt and pepper, if needed. Before serving, top with parsley.

Recipe #36 - Sautéed Cabbage with Corned Beef

Ingredients:

- 3 lbs Corned Beef Brisket

- 1 Green Cabbage, cut into wedges

- 1 medium Onion, wedged

- 1 clove Garlic, chopped finely

Directions:

1. Unpack corned beef brisket and set aside juice and spices. Trim excess fats from beef and place on a 4-quart Dutch oven. Add reserved juice and spices. Add cold water, just enough to cover the meat. Add onion and garlic.

2. Turn heat to high until water starts to boil. Reduce heat to low. Stir and cover. Simmer for 3 hours or until beef is soft and tender.

3. Remove beef and transfer to a warm platter. Keep it warm.

4. Scoop fat from broth. Add cabbage and simmer without cover for 15 minutes or until the cabbage is well cooked.

5. Scoop broth with cabbage in a bowl. Add beef. Serve.

Recipe #37 - Chicken Pot Stickers

Ingredients:

- 1 1/2lbs Chicken, ground
- ½ cup green cabbage, shredded
- 4 medium green onions, chopped
- 1 small red bell pepper, chopped finely
- 2 teaspoons gingerroot, chopped
- ¼ teaspoon white pepper, ground
- 1 teaspoon sesame oil
- 4 teaspoons soy sauce
- 1 large egg white
- 2 cups chicken broth
- 1 10oz pack round wonton skins

Directions:

1. In a large mixing bowl, mix together all ingredients except broth, soy sauce and Wonton skins. Set aside.

2. Lightly brush each Wonton skin with water. Scoop about 1 tablespoon chicken mixture and place in on the middle of each Wonton skin.

3. Pinch 5 pleats on the edge of the other side of the Wonton skin. Close the skin by pressing the unpleated side on the pleated side, folding the skin over the chicken mixture. By now, you should have made a half circle shape with pleats on the edges.

4. Repeat the process until all chicken mixture is used up.

5. Spray a 12-inch skillet with cooking spray and heat over medium temperature. Place 12 pot stickers in the skillet and cook until golden brown. Carefully turn to the other side and cook for another 3 minutes.

6. Add ½ cup chicken broth and 1 teaspoon soy sauce. Cover and cook for 5 minutes over medium heat. Uncover and simmer until liquid evaporates.

7. Repeat the process until all pot stickers are cooked.

Recipe #38 - Fried Broccoli

Ingredients:

- 1/2 cup breadcrumbs
- 1 bunch broccoli, sliced into bite-size cuts
- 1 to 2 tbsps. olive oil
- A pinch rosemary
- Salt and white pepper

Directions:

1. Heat olive oil in a fry pan.

2. Sprinkle with rosemary and sauté until pungent.

3. Sauté broccoli. Season with up to four dashes of white pepper. Continue sautéing broccoli until vibrant green and crunchy.

4. Sprinkle breadcrumbs in batches. Toss and sauté until crumbs start to stick on the vegetable.

5. Once most crumb have already stick, cook for up to 2 minutes more to brown crumbs.

Recipe #39 - Cabbage with Cheese

Ingredients:

- 4 cups Cabbage, chopped
- 1 cup Cheddar Cheese, grated
- 1 cup Milk
- ¾ cup Bread Crumbs
- 3 tablespoons almond flour
- 3 tablespoons Vegetable Oil
- 2 tablespoons Butter, melted
- ½ teaspoon Salt
- A dash of Pepper

Directions:

1. Preheat oven to 350°F. Grease a 2-quart casserole and place cabbage inside. Set aside.

2. Heat saucepan over medium heat and add oil. Add flour, pepper and salt. Cook until bubbles start to appear.

3. Slowly mix in milk and cook until mixture is thick. Add cheese and simmer for 1 minute, stirring from time to time.

4. Pour milk and cheese mixture over cabbage in casserole.

5. In a bowl, mix together bread crumbs and melted butter. Sprinkle on top of cabbage.

6. Bake uncovered for 25 to 30 minutes or until sauce is bubbly.

Recipe #40 - Cheesy Chicken Enchiladas

Ingredients:

- 1 18.5oz can chicken and cheese enchilada soup

- 1 10oz can hot or mild enchilada sauce

- 2 cups cooked chicken, shredded

- 2 cups Monterey jack cheese, shredded

- 10 corn tortillas

- 2 medium green onions, sliced thinly

Directions

1. Preheat oven to 350°F. Grease an 11x7 inches baking pan. Combine enchilada soup and enchilada sauce in a bowl. Pour 1 cup of enchilada sauce mixture into the prepared baking pan and spread evenly.

2. Mix together 1 cup cheese, 1 cup enchilada sauce mixture and chicken in a large bowl. Set aside remaining enchilada sauce mixture.

3. Stack tortillas in a microwaveable plate. Put paper towels on top to cover tortillas. Set microwave to high and heat for 1 minute or until tortillas are soft.

4. Add chicken mixture in the middle of each tortilla. Roll and place on the baking dish with sauce, seams facing down.

5. Drizzle the remaining enchilada sauce mixture over the enchiladas. Spread top with cheese. Garnish with green onions.

6. Bake for 30 minutes or until bubbly on the sides and cheese is melted.

Recipe #41 - Creole-style Cabbage Rolls

Ingredients:

Main Ingredients

- 1 head cabbage, cored and scalded in hot water until tender and easy to set apart
- 2 teaspoon unsalted butter
- 1 cup yellow onions, chopped
- 2 teaspoons garlic, chopped
- ½ lb beef, ground
- ½ lb pork, ground
- 1 cup cooked white rice
- ½ teaspoon salt
- ¼ teaspoon black pepper, ground
- 1 egg

Creole seasoning:

- 2 tablespoons garlic powder
- 2 ½ tablespoons paprika
- 1 tablespoon onion powder
- 1 tablespoon black pepper
- 1 tablespoon cayenne powder
- 1 tablespoon dried thyme
- 1 tablespoon dried oregano leaf

- 2 tablespoons salt

Sauce:

- 2 teaspoons butter

- 1 cup yellow onions, chopped

- 1 teaspoon garlic, minced

- 1 28oz can chopped tomatoes (save the juice)

- 1 cup cream

- 1 tablespoon apple cider vinegar

- 1 tablespoon sugar

Directions:

1. Preheat oven to 350°F.

2. Meanwhile, melt butter in a saucepan over medium heat. Sauté onions and garlic until tender and aromatic. Stir in tomatoes and cream and cook for 5 minutes, stirring occasionally.

3. Stir in vinegar and sugar until mixture thickens. Remove from heat and season with salt and pepper if desired. Set aside

4. Set apart the cabbage leaves and remove the hard middle part on each of them. Pat dry with paper towel. Set aside.

5. On a medium skillet, melt the unsalted butter over medium heat. Add onions and keep mixing until very wilted and butter starts to caramelize.Stir in garlic and cook until aromatic or golden brown. Remove from heat and cool a bit.

6. In a small bowl, combine all ingredients for the essence.

7. In a large mixing bowl, combine pork, beef, rice, egg, Essence, pepper, salt and caramelized onion. You may use your hands or a heavy wooden spoon to mix the ingredients well.

8. On a flat working surface, spread the cabbage leaves with the rib side facing down. Fill the middle of each cabbage leaf with ¼ cup or more meat mixture, depending on how big the leaf is. Roll each leaf into a cylinder.

9. Spread some sauce on the baking dish, evenly distributing on all sides. Line the cabbage rolls on the baking dish with sauce. Repeat the same process until all ingredients are used. Pour top of the rolls with the remaining sauce. Tightly cover with aluminum foil and bake for 2 hours or until meat is properly cooked and cabbage rolls are tender.

10. Line rolls on a serving plate and drizzle some sauce on top.

11. Store the remaining Essence in an airtight container for later use.

Recipe #42 - Grilled Chicken Salad

Ingredients:

- 1 ¼ lb skinless chicken breasts, deboned

- 6 cups assorted salad greens, bite size pieces

- 1 cup strawberries, sliced

- ½ cup frozen non-alcoholic margarita mix, thawed

- ¼ cup cilantro, chopped

- ¼ cup olive oil

- 2 tablespoons white wine vinegar

- 1 medium avocado, pitted, peeled and cubed

- 1 medium mango, pitted, peeled and cubed

Directions:

1. Preheat gas grill or coal grill.

2. Meanwhile, combine margarita mix, vinegar and oil in a small bowl. Mix using a wire whisker until well combined.

3. Baste chicken using ¼ cup salad dressing. Set aside the remaining salad dressing for later use.

4. Grill chicken for 15 to 20 minutes over medium heat, cover. Turn and brush chicken from time to time with ¼ cup salad dressing. Repeat this process until juice that comes out of the chicken is no longer pink when the thickest parts are cut.

5. Slice chicken. In a large salad bowl, toss strawberries, salad greens and chicken. Equally divide among 4 plates. Design each salad plate with avocado and mango pieces. Garnish with cilantro. Drizzle top with remaining salad dressing.

Recipe #43 - Broccoli Quiche

Ingredients

- 4 eggs, well beaten
- 2 cups fresh broccoli, chopped
- 1 onion, chopped finely
- 1 1/2 cups cheese, grated
- 1 1/2 cups skim evaporated milk
- 2 garlic cloves, minced
- 2 tbsps. butter
- 1 pie shell, unbaked
- Salt and pepper

Directions:

1. Preheat oven to 350 degrees F.
2. Melt butter on a large saucepan over medium heat.
3. Sauté garlic, onion and broccoli. Cook slowly while stirring occasionally until tender.
4. Transfer cooked veggies into pie shell.
5. Top with cheese.
6. Mix milk and eggs. Season with salt and pepper.
7. Pour milk mixture on vegetable and cheese layer.
8. Bake for 30 minutes.

Recipe#44 - Japanese-Style Chicken Wings

Ingredients

- 3 pounds chicken wings
- 1 egg, lightly beaten
- 1 cup butter
- 1 cup all-purpose flour for coating

For the Sauce

- 3 tablespoons soy sauce
- 3 tablespoons water
- 1 cup white sugar
- 1/2 cup white vinegar
- 1/2 teaspoon garlic powder, or to taste
- 1 teaspoon salt

Directions:

1. Preheat the oven to 350 degrees F.
2. Prepare a small bowl, beat 1 egg and set aside.
3. In a flat dish, add the flour for dredging and place next to the egg wash.
4. On a chopping board, cut the chicken wings, dip in the egg wash and dredge with flour.
5. In a skillet, melt butter and fry all the chicken wings and transfer to a roasting pan.
6. In a small bowl, add water, sugar, garlic powder, soy sauce, salt, vinegar and salt, pour over the chicken.

7. Transfer the roasting pan in the oven and bake for 45 minutes.

8. Open the oven every 5 minutes to baste the chicken with the sauce.

9. Once the chicken is done, serve the Japanese-style chicken wings on a plate and serve.

Recipe #45 - Eggplant Parmigiana

Ingredients:

- 1/2 cup Parmigiano-Reggiano, freshly grated
- 2 large eggplants, (approximately 2 pounds)
- 2 cups of basic tomato sauce, recipe is below
- olive oil, extra-virgin
- Salt and pepper
- 1 bunch of chiffonade basil leaves, fresh
- 1 pound of mozzarella cheese, fresh, sliced to 1/8-inch thick pieces
- 1/4 cup of bread crumbs, fresh and lightly toasted under broiler

For the basic tomato sauce:

- 1 Spanish onion, diced into 1/4-inch pieces
- 1/4 cup olive oil, extra-virgin
- 3 tablespoons of chopped fresh thyme, or 1 tablespoon if dried
- 4 cloves of garlic, peeled and then thinly sliced
- 1/2 carrot, medium, finely grated
- Salt
- 2 (28-ounce) cans of peeled whole tomatoes

Directions

1. For the tomato sauce: Crush peeled whole tomatoes by hand and then set juices aside.
2. Heat olive oil in a 3-quart saucepan over heat set at medium. Add in the garlic and onion. Cook until onions are soft and

turn a light golden brown, which should take about 8 minutes.

3. Add the carrot and thyme and then cook for an additional 5 minutes, or until carrot is pretty soft. Then, add tomatoes and the juice you set aside. Bring mixture to a boil while stirring often.

4. Reduce heat. Simmer for about 30 minutes or until consistency is thick and resembles hot cereal.

5. Season sauce with salt.

6. For the Parmigiana Preheat oven to a temperature of 450 degrees F.

7. Grease a baking sheet with some extra-virgin olive oil

8. Cut each of the eggplants into 6 disks, resulting to slices that are from 1-inch to 1 1/2 inches thick. Season each disk lightly with salt and pepper. Place on the greased sheet and then at a temperature of 450 degrees F for around 12-15 minutes, or until the slices begin to turn deep brown on top.

9. remove eggplants from oven. Get slices off the baking sheet and transfer to a plate. Allow to cool.

10. Reduce the oven's temperature to 350 degrees F. Place the 4 largest eggplant slices in an 8x12 (inches) brownie pan, making sure they are evenly spaced apart. Spread 1/4 cup of tomato sauce over each slice, and then sprinkle with about a teaspoon of basil.

11. Place one slice of mozzarella cheese over each slice and then sprinkle with a teaspoon of Parmigiano. Then, place smaller eggplant slices on top of the larger disks and repeat the layering process, toping with the tomato sauce, and then basil, followed with the 2 cheeses. Keep on doing the layering until ingredients are used up.

12. Top the eggplant dish with toasted bread crumbs and then bake uncovered for around 20 minutes, or just until the cheese melts and you see that the tops are light brown. Serve immediately.

Recipe #46 - Chicken Salad Veronique

Ingredients

- 4 split chicken breasts

- 1 cup green grapes, halved

- 1 cup celery, diced

- ½ cup mayonnaise

- 1 ½ tablespoons tarragon leaves, chopped

- olive oil

- salt

- ground black pepper

Directions

1. Preheat oven to 350°F.

2. Rub each chicken meat with olive oil. Season each side with salt and pepper.

3. Oven roast for 35 to 40 minutes or until chicken is cooked through and through. Cool.

4. Separate bone and skin from chicken meat. Discard skin and bones.

5. Dice chicken meat into ¾-inch pieces.

6. In a bowl, combine chicken meat, mayonnaise, celery, tarragon leaves and grapes. Toss to blend all ingredients. Season with salt and pepper.

7. Chill for an hour and serve.

Recipe #47 – Asian-Style Chicken Wings

Ingredients:

- 1 teaspoon salt
- 5 pounds chicken wings
- 1 tablespoon mixed spices seasoning
- 2 cups fresh orange juice
- 2 tablespoons garlic, minced
- 1/2 teaspoon ground white pepper
- 1 cup sugar
- 1 cup pineapple juice
- 2 tablespoons fresh ginger, minced
- 2 tablespoons orange zest
- 1/2 cup soy sauce
- 2 tablespoons green onions, minced
- 1 tablespoon sesame oil
- 1/2 cup rice wine, non-alcoholic
- 2 tablespoons sliced green onions, for garnish
- 3/4 teaspoon red pepper, crushed
- 2 tablespoons sesame seeds

Directions:

1. Preheat oven to 425 degrees F and line a baking sheet with aluminum foil.
2. In a medium-sized bowl, rub the chicken wings with mixed spices seasoning.

3. Transfer the chicken wings in the baking sheet, place in the oven and bake for 35 minutes.

4. Meanwhile, in a large skillet, prepare the sauce by adding the rest of the remaining ingredients except the green onions and sesame seeds.

5. Bring to a rolling boil; constantly stir the ingredients until the syrup is formed, remove chicken from the heat.

6. As soon as the timer stops at 35 minutes, remove the wings from the oven and reduce the temperature to 350 degrees F.

7. Transfer the cooked wings into a bowl, drizzle half of the sauce and sprinkle sesame seeds.

8. Place the chicken back into the oven and bake for 25 minutes or until it cooks through.

9. Serve the chicken wings on a platter and garnish with sliced green onions.

Recipe #48 - Ground Beef in Mushroom Sauce

Ingredients:

- 1 ½ pounds ground sirloin
- 4 cups sliced mushrooms
- 1 small diced onion
- ½ cup heavy cream
- 2 tablespoons chopped parsley
- 2 tablespoons vegetable oil
- Salt and pepper

Directions:

1. Combine sirloin, salt and pepper. Mix well. Form 4 patties.

2. Heat the oil on a skillet on medium high heat. Cook patties for 5 minutes or until brown.

3. Leave about 1 tablespoon fat from the skillet. Add onion and cook for 2 minutes until soft.

4. Add mushrooms and continue cooking until mushrooms are soft and have given off liquid. This will take about 10 minutes.

5. Stir in cream and wait for it to thicken for about 2 minutes.

6. Add parsley.

7. Return the patties to the skillet. Coat the patties in sauce for 3 minutes.

8. Spoon the mushrooms on top and serve.

Recipe #49 - Glazed Meatloaves

Ingredients:

- 1 ½ pounds ground meat (combination of ground beef, ground pork and ground turkey)
- 17-20 crushed saltine crackers
- 1/3 cup minced fresh parsley
- ¼ cup whole milk
- 1 egg
- 3 tablespoons Worcestershire sauce
- 1 ½ tablespoons Dijon mustard
- 1 teaspoon garlic powder
- 1 teaspoon onion powder
- Salt and pepper
- 2 teaspoons canola oil

Glaze:

- ¼ cup stevia
- ½ cup ketchup
- 4 teaspoons cider vinegar

Directions:

1. Heat the oven to 425 degrees Fahrenheit.

2. Mix saltine cracker crumbs, parsley, milk, egg, mustard, Worcestershire sauce, garlic powder, onion powder, salt and pepper in a mixing bowl. Mix in ground meat.

3. Mold the mixture into oval loaves.

4. Heat oil in a skillet on medium heat. Add meatloaves and brown for 3-5 minutes. Flip and brown for another 2-3 minutes.

5. Mix glaze ingredients until smooth.

6. Transfer mini meatloaves to a baking pan and place glaze over the top of each meatloaf. Bake for 18-20 minutes until the temperature of the center of the meatloaf is 160 degrees.

Recipe #50 - Broccoli with Garlic and Lemon

Ingredients:

- 2 broccoli heads, peel stems and cut heads into half lengthwise
- 3 tbsps. extra virgin olive oil
- 3 garlic cloves, sliced thinly
- 2 tbsps. fresh lemon juice
- 1/2 cup water
- 1 pinch crushed red pepper
- Salt and black pepper

Directions:

1. Heat 2 tablespoons of oil into a deep pan.
2. Place broccoli on the pan with cut side down. Cover and cook over medium heat for 8 minutes until browned.
3. Pour water. Cook for 7 minutes until broccoli is tender.
4. Add another tablespoon of oil into the pan.
5. Add crushed red pepper and garlic. Cook without covering for 3 minutes.
6. Season with freshly ground black pepper and salt.
7. Drizzle with lemon juice before serving.

Recipe #51 - Three-Cheese Eggplant

Ingredients:

- 1 beaten egg
- 1 pound angel hair pasta
- 1 peeled eggplant, slices lengthwise into 1/4 inch pieces
- 1 cup of bread crumbs seasoned with Italian seasoning
- 1 cup of ricotta cheese
- 2 tablespoons of olive oil
- 10 slices of prosciutto
- 1 (14 ounce) jar of spaghetti sauce
- 2 cups mozzarella cheese, shredded

Directions:

1. Dip eggplant slices in egg, and then coat with the bread crumbs.

2. In a large pan over moderate-high heat, heat the olive oil, and then fry eggplant slices on each side until they turn golden brown. Transfer to a plate lined with paper towel to remove excess oil.

3. Preheat oven to a temperature of 350 degrees F.

4. Spread just a thin layer of ricotta onto each eggplant slice, and then place a prosciutto slice on top. Tightly roll up the slices. Place with the seam of the rolls facing down into a 9 by 13 (inches) baking dish.

5. Pour the spaghetti sauce over the eggplant rolls. Top with mozzarella cheese and then bake in preheated oven for about 15 minutes, or until the cheese has been melted and has turned lightly brown.

6. Prepare the pasta while rolls are baking. Place water in a large pot, add a small amount of salt and then bring to a boil. Add angel hair pasta, and then cook for about 2 to 3 minutes, or until tender, and then drain.

7. Serve the eggplant rolls and sauce over the pasta.

Recipe #52 - Pork Chop and Broccoli Bake

Ingredients:

- 6 pork chops, bone-in, half-inch thick

- 1 11-oz. can condensed Cheddar cheese soup

- 3 cups fresh broccoli florets, chopped

- 1 20-oz. bag cooked shredded hash browns, refrigerated

- 1/2 cup each of milk and sour cream

- 1 tbsp. olive oil

- 1 onion, medium, chopped

- Salt and pepper

Directions:

1. Preheat oven (350 degrees Fahrenheit). Mix the dairy ingredients, potatoes, onions and broccoli in a large mixing bowl. Transfer mixture into an ungreased 13 x 9-inch glass oven dish. Cover then bake for 30 minutes

2. While baking, heat oil in a pan over medium heat. Fry three pork chops and season with salt and pepper. Cook each side for 3 to 5 minutes or until brown. Do the same procedures for the remaining chops.

3. Take the oven dish out and remove lid. Top the baked mixture with pork chops. Bake for 25 minutes or more as long as pork is cooked through or when edges are bubbly.

Recipe #53 - Spicy Buffalo Chicken Wings

Ingredients

- 10 chicken wings
- 1/4 teaspoon paprika
- 1/2 cup all-purpose flour
- Oil (for deep frying)
- 1/4 cup hot sauce
- 1/4 teaspoon salt
- 1/4 teaspoon cayenne pepper
- 1/4 cup butter
- 1 dash garlic powder
- 1 dash ground black pepper

Directions:

1. In a small bowl, mix paprika, black pepper, flour, salt and cayenne pepper.
2. In a glass dish, place the chicken wings.
3. Add the flour mixture until the wings are full covered.
4. Once the wings are coated, refrigerate the dish for an hour.
5. After an hour, preheat your deep fryer to 375 degrees F.
6. Fill the fryer with oil and add the refrigerated chicken wings.
7. In a saucepan, add butter then combine the butter and garlic powder; cook under low heat.
8. Once the chicken has turned golden brown, transfer them on a plate and coat with the spicy butter sauce.
9. Serve with sour cream and cilantro for dipping.

Recipe #54 - Roasted Broccoli

Ingredients:

- 1 large head broccoli, cut into florets and stems, set a quarter-inch thickness

- 2 tsps. fresh lemon juice

- 1/4 cup extra virgin olive oil

- 1 1/2 tbsps. pine nuts

- 1 tsp. shallots, minced

- Basil leaves thinly sliced

- Salt and black pepper

Directions

1. Preheat oven (400 degrees Fahrenheit).

2. Spread broccoli on a baking sheet.

3. Drizzle broccoli with 2 tablespoons olive oil. toss well to coat each piece

4. Roast for 30 minutes in the oven until tender and brown. Toss halfway.

5. Set a pan over medium heat and toast nuts for 4 minutes until golden.

6. Combine shallots, juice and 2 tablespoons oil in a small bowl. Season with freshly ground pepper and salt.

7. Take out the baking sheet and transfer broccoli in a serving bowl.

8. Drizzle with dressing. Top with basil and nuts. Toss well to coat.

Recipe #55 - Grilled Tuna

Ingredients:

- 3 tuna steaks, 4 oz each

- 2 Tbsp. olive oil

- 1 ½ Tbsp. fresh cilantro, minced

- 1 ½ Tbsp. fresh Italian parsley, minced

- 4 garlic cloves, minced

- 1/3 tsp sea salt

- ¼ tsp paprika

- 1 small lemon

Directions:

1. Combine the herbs with the salt, paprika, and garlic. Juice and zest the lemon, then add to the mixture. Stir in the olive oil.

2. Place the tuna steaks in a baking dish and add the mixture. Turn to coat, then cover and refrigerate for 1 hour.

3. After marinating, set the grill to medium high flame.

4. Grill the tuna steaks for 3 to 4 minutes per side, basting with the marinade.

5. Let rest for 5 minutes before serving.

Recipe #56 - Pot Roast

Ingredients:

- 3 to 5-lb. chuck roast, one whole meat

- 6 to 8 carrots, unpeeled, cut into 4-cm pieces

- 2 onions, peeled and cut into half

- 3 cups beef stock

- 2 to 3 tbsps. olive oil

- 2 to 3 sprigs each of fresh thyme and fresh rosemary

- Salt and pepper

- 1 cup red wine, optional

Directions:

1. Preheat oven (275 degrees Fahrenheit). Season meat with salt and pepper. Heat oil in a Dutch oven or big pot over medium heat. Add onions and cook until sides are brown. Transfer to a plate.

2. Cook carrots on the same pot for a minute. Toss lightly until it browns in color. Set it beside onions once done. Add more oil if needed for cooking meat. Put chuck roast inside the pot and sear until all sides are brown. Transfer roast on a plate.

3. Use a cup of beef stock or red wine to remove glaze from the pot. Don't reduce the burner's heat. Scrape and whisk the bottom part of the pan. Place the meat back into the pot and pour the remaining stock or add enough just to cover it halfway. Add carrots, onions and fresh herbs.

4. Cover the pot and cook for 3 hours for every 3-pound meat. Cook for 4 hours if the meat weighs 4 to 5 pounds. Continue

cooking until meat is very tender that it's falling apart with a slight nudge.

Recipe#57 - Asian-Style Eggplant

Ingredients:

- 4 tablespoons of vegetable oil (to be divided into 2 tablespoons each)
- 4 Japanese eggplants, cubed into 1-inch cuts
- 2 onions, medium, thinly sliced
- 2 tablespoons soy sauce
- 1 tablespoon garlic, minced
- 2 tablespoons of water
- 1 tablespoon of chili-garlic sauce
- 1 1/2 tablespoons of oyster sauce
- 1 teaspoon of white sugar
- 1/2 teaspoon toasted sesame oil, Asian style
- black pepper, freshly ground to taste

Directions:

1. In a large wok or skillet, heat 2 tablespoons of oil over medium-high heat settings until it's almost smoking.

2. Add eggplant cubes, stirring for 3 to 5 minutes or until they start to turn. Use a slotted spoon to remove eggplant slices. Set aside.

3. In the skillet, heat what's left of the oil over medium-high heat, and then cook the onions, constantly stirring just until the point that they begin to get tender, which should take about 30 seconds. Then, stir in the minced garlic. Cook and stir for 30 seconds more and then add in the water, soy sauce, oyster sauce, sugar, black pepper, and chili garlic sauce. Stir until a smooth sauce forms.

4. Return eggplant slices to the skillet, and then reduce heat. Let sauce and vegetables to simmer until the eggplant slices are

tender and almost all of the sauce is absorbed, which should take about 5 minutes. Drizzle sesame oil, and then give stir briefly for one last time to combine.

Recipe #58 - Baked Sausage Balls

Ingredients:

- 1 package cheddar cheese
- Vegetable oil
- 1 lb. beef or pork sausage
- Bottled Mustard dip
- 2 cups multi-purpose baking mix
- Fresh Cilantro leaves, for garnishing

Directions:

1. Preheat your oven to 400 degrees F.

2. In a mixing bowl, add the multi-purpose flour baking mix, water and cheese.

3. In a cookie sheet, line aluminum foil and coat it with vegetable oil.

4. After making the dough, roll it to a ball and put the sliced sausages in the middle and pop it in the oven for 12 minutes.

5. When the sausage roll is done, remove from the cookie sheet and drain excess oil on a paper towel.

6. Serve with a mustard dip and garnish with cilantro.

Recipe #59 - Mushroom Sausage Stuffing

Ingredients:

- 3/4 pound sweet Italian sausage

- 2 and 1/2 tablespoons Marsala wine

- Pepper

- 16 white extra-large mushrooms

- 5 tablespoons olive oil

- 2/3 cup breadcrumbs

- 6 scallions

- 5 ounces mascarpone cheese

- 2 1/2 tablespoons fresh parsley leaves

- 2 garlic cloves

- 1/3 cup Parmesan cheese

- Salt

Directions:

1. Preheat the oven to 325 degrees F.

2. In a shallow bowl, add whole mushroom caps, Marsala wine and olive oil.

3. If you cannot find the Marsala wine, you can substitute it with brandy or sherry wine.

4. In a medium-sized skillet, add 2 tbsp. of olive oil and cook the sausages for 8 minutes.

5. Crumble the cooked sweet Italian sausages and stir in the garlic, breadcrumbs, mascarpone and scallions.

6. Once they are combined, add the Parmesan cheese, pepper, salt and parsley leaves.

7. Take the mushroom caps and fill its center with the cooked sausage and garlic mixture.

8. Line the mushrooms in a greased baking dish and bake for 50 minutes.

9. Once the stuffing has turned golden brown, turn off the heat to serve the Marsala Sausage Mushroom Stuffing.

Recipe #60 - Baked Pork Chops

Ingredients:

- 6 pork chops

- 2 cups seasoned bread crumbs, Italian-style

- 1 can condensed cream of mushroom soup, 10.75 oz.

- 2 eggs, beaten

- 1/3 cup white wine

- 1/4 cup all-purpose flour

- 1/2 cup milk

- 4 tbsps. olive oil

- 1 tsp. each of garlic powder and seasoning salt

Directions:

1. Preheat oven (350 degrees Fahrenheit). Rinse meat then pat dry using paper towels or clean towel. Season with salt and garlic powder according to preferred taste.

2. Prepare three shallow dishes or platter. Put eggs in one dish, bread crumbs on the other, and flour on the last dish. Get seasoned pork and dredge in flour and shake excess back to the platter. Dip on eggs then coat with bread crumbs.

3. Heat oil in a pan. Cook chops for 5 minutes on each side or until they are brown. Arrange pre-cooked meat in a 9 x 13-inch oven dish then cover. Bake for an hour.

4. While baking combine the remaining liquid ingredients in a bowl. Pour the mixture over baked meat after the first hour. Cover again then continue baking for 30 minutes.

Recipe #61 - Spicy Halibut

Ingredients:

- 3 boneless halibut fillets, 4 oz each

- 2 ½ Tbsp extra virgin olive oil

- 3 garlic cloves, minced

- 1 red chili pepper, minced

- 1 ½ cups seedless green grapes

- ¼ cup torn fresh basil leaves

- Sea salt

- Freshly ground black pepper

Directions:

1. Pour the olive oil in a cast iron skillet over medium high flame.

2. Lay the halibut into the skillet, then add the garlic, chili pepper, basil, and grapes. Season lightly with salt and pepper.

3. Add 1 cup of water, then reduce to medium low flame. Cover and cook for 7 minutes per side, or until the fish is cooked through. Transfer the halibut to a platter.

4. Simmer the sauce over high flame until slightly thickened. Adjust seasoning, if needed. Pour over the fish.

Recipe #62 - Seafood in Tomato Sauce

Ingredients:

- 2 Tbsp olive oil

- ¾ lb medium shrimp, peeled and deveined

- 12 mussels, scrubbed and debearded

- ½ small red onion, minced

- 2 small garlic cloves, crushed

- 3 ripe tomatoes

- ½ cup chopped fresh basil

- ¼ cup chopped fresh oregano

- 1/3 cup dry white wine

- Sea salt

- Freshly ground black pepper

Directions:

1. Puree the tomatoes in a food processor. Set aside.

2. Place a saucepan over medium flame and add 1 tablespoon of olive oil. Sauté the onion and garlic until tender, then add the pureed tomatoes and season with salt and pepper to taste.

3. Reduce to low flame and cover the pot. Simmer for 1o minutes or until thickened.

4. Stir in the herbs and simmer for 5 minutes, then turn off the heat.

5. Meanwhile, pour the wine into a nonreactive pot and add the mussels. Place over high flame and bring to a boil.

6. Once boiling, reduce to a simmer and steam the mussels for 7 minutes, or until they open. Discard unopened mussels, then drain.

7. Place a cast iron skillet over high flame and add the remaining olive oil. Cook the shrimp for 2 minutes per side or until cooked through. Add the steamed mussels and sauté to combine.

8. Pour in the tomato sauce and mix well. Cover and simmer for 3 minutes, then serve with brown rice or crusty bread.

CHAPTER 4 KETO DINNER RECIPES

Recipe #63 - Sweet and Spicy Shrimp

Ingredients:

- ¾ lb peeled and deveined large shrimp, uncooked
- ½ green bell pepper, cut into pieces
- 1 tbsp vegetable oil
- ½ tsp crushed red pepper
- ½ tsp sesame oil
- 1 medium carrot, thinly sliced
- 1 onion, cut into pieces
- 2 tsp cornstarch
- 2 tsp sugar
- ¼ cup soy sauce

Directions:

1. Let shrimp thaw (if needed).

2. Combine the sesame oil, crushed red pepper, sugar, soy sauce and cornstarch in a bowl. Stir until the ingredients are fully dissolved. Set it aside.

3. Pour the oil in a large pan. Place it over medium heat. Sauté the bell pepper, carrot and onion for 3 minutes until it is crispy tender.

4. Combine the shrimp and soy sauce mixture. Stir for 5 minutes and cook until the shrimps are pink and the sauce is thick. Serve with rice if desired.

Recipe #64 - Lemon- Garlic Shrimp

Ingredients:

- 2 tbsp fresh parsley, roughly chopped

- Pinch of cayenne pepper

- 1 lb shrimp, peeled, deveined

- ¼ cup grated parmesan cheese

- ¾ cup instant grits

- 2 large garlic cloves, minced

- 2 tbsp unsalted butter

- Salt and pepper to taste

- Juice of half lemon and lemon wedges for serving

Directions:

1. Boil 3 cups of water in a pan over medium heat. Uncover and whisk in the grits. ½ tsp pepper 1 tsp salt. Simmer and stir the mixture occasionally until the liquid is thick. Stir in the parmesan with the 1 tbsp butter. Remove it from the heat. Season with the salt and pepper. Cover and keep warm.

2. Season the shrimp with salt and pepper. Melt the remaining butter in a pan. Add the garlic, shrimp and cayenne. Cook the shrimp for 4 minutes. Remove from the heat.

3. Add 2 tbsp water, parsley and lemon juice. Toss to coat the shrimp with the sauce. Adjust the seasoning if needed.

4. Divide it into bowls. Top with the sauce and shrimp. Garnish with lemon wedges before serving.

Recipe #65 - Sausage and Vegetable Soup

Ingredients:

- 2 small zucchini
- 1 clove garlic
- 1 green pepper
- 5 cups chicken broth
- 2 carrots
- Ground pepper
- 2/3 cup freshly grated parmesan cheese
- 1/2 cup dry white wine
- 1 medium onion
- 1/2 teaspoon dried oregano
- 1 can crushed tomatoes puree
- 1 lb. Italian sausage
- 1 teaspoon dried basil
- Salt
- 1/2 cup uncooked rice-shaped pasta

Directions:

1. In a large saucepan, cook the bulk sausage without the casing then add pepper, dry white wine, chicken broth, tomatoes, basil, carrots, oregano and zucchini then bring all ingredients to a boil.

2. When the saucepan has reached a boil, add the uncooked rice-shaped pasta and cook for about 20 minutes.

3. Transfer the soup to a large bowl and serve while hit.

Recipe #66 – Caribbean-Style Chicken Salad

Ingredients:

Dressing

- 1 6oz container fat-free pina colada yogurt
- 2 tablespoons lime juice
- 1 teaspoon dry caribbean jerk seasoning

Salad

- 3 cups romaine lettuce, shredded
- 2 cups cooked chicken, cubed
- 1 cup ripe mango, diced
- 1 cup monterey jack cheese, shredded
- 1 cup cheddar cheese, shredded
- ½ cup plum tomatoes, seeded and chopped
- ½ cup green onions, sliced thinly
- ½ cup cashews

Directions:

1. Mix all dressing ingredients together in a bowl until well blended.

2. In a clear glass serving bowl, layer the salad ingredients according to the list. Leave the cashews.

3. Drizzle dressing on top of salad and garnish with cashews.

Recipe #67 - Cheese Broccoli Soup

Ingredients:

- 2 cups milk

- Two 10.75-oz. cans chicken stock

- 1 bunch broccoli

- 1/2 cup flour

- 1/2 cup butter

- 1 cup sharp or mild cheddar cheese, grated

- 1 onion, medium, chopped

- Velveeta cheese

- Salt and pepper

Directions:

1. Cook broccoli until tender. Drain and set aside. Melt butter and sauté onions until translucent and tender.

2. Add flour and stir. Cook for 5 minutes and stir constantly. Pour milk gradually while stirring constantly.

3. Add grated cheese and cook until smooth. Pour broth gradually the stir. Blend well until smooth.

4. Add Velveeta cheese. Cook until it melts. Divide cooked broccoli. Puree half using a food processor or a fork.

5. Slice the remaining broccoli into small pieces. Stir broccoli into the soup.

6. Cook and simmer for 15 minutes.

Recipe #68 – Keto-Style Chicken Salad

Ingredients:

- 1 large egg

- A cup of spinach

- 2 cups of shredded chicken breast meat

- 2 rashers of bacon

- 2 tablespoons of avocado

- Half a teaspoon of white vinegar

- A tablespoon of olive oil

Directions:

1. Hard boil an egg for about 10 minutes. Cool the egg and then peel and chop the egg. Set aside.

2. Fry the bacon according to your preference.

3. On another pan, cook the shredded chicken breast until done.

4. Once chicken breast is cooked, remove pan from direct heat.

5. Add the chopped eggs into the pan.

6. Rip or chop spinach leaves to smaller pieces and add pieces into the pan.

7. Add the avocado in the pan. Mix thoroughly until avocado breaks into smaller pieces.

8. Dress the salad with some vinegar and olive oil. Serve.

Recipe #69 – Chicken and Bacon Roll

Ingredients:

- 1 large chicken breast, slice into small bite size portions
- 9 slices of bacon cut into thirds
- 3 tablespoons of garlic powder

Directions:

1. Preheat oven to 205C. Line a baking tray with some aluminum foil.

2. Coat each chicken piece with some garlic powder.

3. Wrap bacon around each chicken piece and secure with a toothpick.

4. Place the bacon wrapped chicken pieces on the baking tray.

5. Bake for 25-30 minutes or until the bacons turns crispy. Turn bacon wrapped pieces after 15 minutes.

Recipe #70 - Onion Cheese Soup

Ingredients:

- 8 oz slices reduced-fat and reduced-sodium Swiss cheese

- ¼ tsp fresh thyme, chopped

- ¼ cup dry white wine

- ½ tsp freshly ground black pepper

- 4 cups red onion, thinly sliced

- 2 tsp olive oil

- 8 oz French bread, cut into cubes

- 8 cups less sodium beef broth

- ½ tsp salt

- ½ tsp sugar

- 4 cups sweet onion, thinly sliced

Directions:

1. Heat olive oil in a Dutch oven. Add the onions and cook until it is tender. Add the pepper, sugar and ¼ tsp salt. Reduce the heat and cook for 20 minutes.

2. Stir the mixture frequently and increase the heat to high. Cook until the onions are golden brown. Add the wine and cook for a minute. Add the thyme and broth. Boil then simmer for 2 hours.

3. Preheat the broiler. Place the bread in a baking sheet. Broil for 2 minutes until it is toasted.

4. Place 8 bowls on a jelly roll pan. Ladle one cup of the soup into each bowl. Place the bread on top and serve with cheese slice. Broil until the cheese begins to brown.

Recipe #71 - Garlic Beef Stroganoff

Ingredients:

- 2 teaspoons of beef bouillon granules
- 2 cups sliced mushrooms
- 1 cup of boiling water
- 1 onion, large chopped
- 1 can condensed cream of mushroom soup
- 3 cloves of garlic, minced
- 1 and 1/2 to 2 pounds of beef top round steak
- 1 tablespoon of Worcestershire sauce
- 1 package (8 ounces) of cream cheese, cubed
- 2 tablespoons of canola oil
- Cooked noodles, hot

Directions:

1. Cut beef into thin strips.

2. Dissolve bouillon granules in water inside a 3-quart slow cooker. Add cream of mushroom, onion, mushrooms, Worcestershire sauce and garlic.

3. In a pan, brown beef in canola oil. Transfer beef to slow cooker and then place lid. Cook on low until the meat is tender, which should take around 7 to 8 hours. Add cream cheese 5 minutes before serving and stir well until smooth. Serve with cooked noodles. This makes 6 to 8 servings.

Recipe #72 - Mushroom Chicken Recipe

Ingredients:

- 170 grams of chicken

- 227 grams of mushrooms

- Water

- Heavy cream

- Fresh lemon juice

- Salt and pepper to taste

- A handful of spinach

Directions:

1. Cook chicken in a pan halfway through. Remove from pan and allow chicken to rest.

2. Add the mushrooms and some butter on the same pan and cook until mushrooms become crispy and shrunken.

3. Mix lemon juice, water and heavy cream in the pan. Cook sauce until it thickens.

4. Season the sauce with some salt and pepper.

5. Put the chicken back into the pan and cook until done.

6. Plate cooked chicken and top with some chopped spinach. Serve.

Recipe #73 - Cheesy Bake Veggies with Mushrooms

Ingredients:

- 2g of olive oil

- 20g of onions, chopped

- 30g of mushrooms, chopped

- 50g of leeks, sliced

- 20g of chicken breast, diced

- 1 portion of the cheese sauce (see recipe for Cauliflower Baked Cheese)

- 10g of parmesan cheese, finely grated

Directions:

1. Preheat oven to 190 degrees.

2. In a pan, heat olive oil and sauté onion until soft and translucent.

3. Mix in leeks, mushrooms, and diced chicken and cook until browned.

4. Mix vegetables, chicken and cheese sauce together and transfer to an oven proof dish.

5. Sprinkle with grated parmesan cheese and bake for approximately 20 minutes or until golden brown and chicken is cooked through.

6. Remove from oven and serve hot.

Recipe #74 – Chicken and Vegetable Soup Recipe

Ingredients:

- 2 tbsp Parmesan cheese, grated

- 2 cups, whole wheat wide noodle pasta

- 2 celery stalks, sliced

- 3 inch Parmesan rind

- 1 ½ lb bone-in chicken breast, skin removed

- 6 3-inch strips lemon zest from 1 lemon

- Pinch crushed red pepper flakes

- 1 tbsp extra virgin olive oil

- 3 cups baby spinach

- Kosher salt

- 2 carrots, sliced

- 8 cups low sodium chicken broth

- 1 small head fennel, thinly sliced

- 6 whole sprigs, plus 1 tbsp flat leaf parsley

- 1 onion, chopped

Directions:

1. Pour oil in a Dutch oven over medium heat. Add the red pepper and onion. Cook until the onions are tender.

2. Tie the parsley sprigs, fennel tops and lemon zest. Add the herbs into a pot. Place the chicken in the pot. Add the cheese

rind and 2 cups of water. Bring to boil then simmer for 8 minutes.

3. Place the chicken into the cutting board and let it cool. Remove the meat from the bones and cut into large strips.

4. Add the celery, sliced fennel and carrots. Season with salt. Simmer until vegetables are crisp-tender. Add the noodles and cook for 5 minutes.

5. Add the reserved chicken, Parmesan rind and baby spinach. Stir in the lemon juice and ladle the soup into bowls. Top with Parmesan if desired.

Recipe #75 - Cheesy Broccoli Soup

Ingredients

- 8 oz light processed cheese, cubed

- ½ cup all purpose flour

- 16 oz packed broccoli florets

- 2 garlic cloves, minced

- ¼ tsp black pepper

- 2 ½ cups 2% fat milk

- 3 cups chicken broth, less sodium

- 1 cup onion, chopped

- Cooking spray

Directions:

1. Place a large pan over medium heat. Coat the bottom with cooking spray. Add garlic and onion. Cook for 3 minutes until tender.

2. Add the broccoli and broth. Boil the mixture at high heat. Cook for 10 minutes.

3. Combine the flour and milk. Whisk until combined. Add the mixture to the broccoli. Cook for 5 minutes until it is thick. Add the pepper and cheese. Continue to cook until the cheese melts

4. Process 1/3 of the mixture in a blender until smooth. Return to the pan and reheat before serving.

Recipe #76 - Fried Spinach

Ingredients:

- 2 cups seasoned bread crumbs
- 2 cups all purpose flour
- 1 ½ cups Parmesan cheese
- 2 cups fresh spinach, chopped
- 3 garlic cloves, minced
- ¼ cup extra virgin olive oil
- 1 ½ cups Arborio rice
- 2 cups chicken broth
- 2 eggs, lightly beaten
- 8 oz mozzarella cheese, cut into cubes
- 2 tbsp butter
- 1 cup white wine
- 1 onion, minced
- Salt and pepper to taste
- ½ tsp saffron threads, crumbled
- Vegetable oil for deep frying

Directions:

1. Combine the chicken broth and saffron threads in a pan and boil at high heat. Stir in the Arborio rice. Simmer until the rice is tender. This usually takes about 16 minutes.

2. Heat the olive oil in a pan. Add the onion and cook for a minute. Add the garlic and cook for 3-4 minutes or until it is translucent and soft.

3. Add the butter, wine and spinach. Boil the mixture and reduce the heat. Add the Parmesan cheese and cooked rice. Cook until the mixture is a little stiff.

4. Spread it over the baking sheet. Place it in the refrigerator for at least 4 hours to overnight until it is completely cold.

5. Form the arancini by placing a cube of mozzarella cheese in the middle of a 1 inch rice ball. Set it aside. Place flour, bread crumbs and eggs in a separate bowls. Roll the arancini in the flour then dip it into the egg. Dip it into the bread crumbs. Repeat the process for all the arancini.

6. Heat oil in a large fryer. Place 5-6 arancini in the pan with oil. Cook the arancini in the oil until it is golden brown. Make sure to roll the arancini to make sure that it cooks evenly. Place over paper towels to absorb excess oil.

Recipe #77 - Spinach Tortellini Soup

Ingredients:

- ¼ cup Parmesan cheese, freshly grated
- Cracked black pepper
- 9 oz pack fresh tortellini
- 4-6 cups chicken broth
- ½ cup onion, minced
- 10 oz fresh spinach
- Kosher salt
- 14 oz can whole tomatoes, coarsely chopped
- 1 garlic clove, minced
- 1 tbsp. olive oil

Directions:

1. Heat the olive oil in a pot.

2. Cook the onion and garlic. Stir it often until it is translucent. This usually takes about 5-7 minutes.

3. Add tomatoes and broth. Increase the heat then boil the mixture.

4. Add the tortellini. Cook it according to the pack instructions.

5. Add the spinach and adjust the seasoning with salt and pepper.

6. Garnish each serving with parmesan cheese before serving.

Recipe #78 - Sausage Cups with Sour Cream

Ingredients:

- 3/4 container sour cream

- 1/2 cup hard cheese (Muenster)

- 1 bunch of scallions

- 1 pound Italian sausage

- 1 cup salsa

- 1/2 cup shredded cheddar cheese

- 24 pieces wonton wrappers

Directions:

1. Preheat your oven to 350 degrees F.

2. In a deep skillet, add crumbled Italian sausages and cook them until golden brown.

3. Once the sausages are done, remove the skillet from the heat and add the hard cheeses.

4. Lightly grease a small muffin pan with olive oil and line it with wonton wrappers.

5. Fill the wrapper with sausage mixture and bake in the oven for 10 minutes.

6. Once the wonton wrappers are done, peel them from the muffin pans and serve on a plate.

7. Garnish each of the Sausage Wonton Cup with sour cream and scallions.

Recipe #79 - Chicken and Spinach Curry

Ingredients:

- 9g of olive oil

- 20g of onions

- 2g of garlic

- 45g of chicken breast

- ½ teaspoon of curry powder

- 20g of mushrooms

- A pinch of salt

- 25g of spinach

- 4g desiccated coconut

Directions:

1. In a pan over medium heat, heat some olive oil.

2. Add the chopped garlic and onions in to the pan and fry until it softens.

3. Add the chicken, the curry powder, mushrooms, and the desiccated coconut. Stir fry everything until chicken turns brown.

4. Allow curry to simmer for 20 minutes before taking pan off the heat.

5. Add the spinach and stir curry.

6. In another frying pan, put the remaining coconut and toast.

7. Before serving, sprinkle some toasted coconut on top of the curry. Serve.

Recipe #80 - Flank Steak (Slow Cooker Recipe)

Ingredients:

- 1 cup beef broth
- 1 tsp salt
- 1 tsp dried oregano leaves
- 1 beef flank steak, cut into 8 pieces
- 1 red bell pepper, cut into strip
- 2 tbsp lime juice
- 2 tsp dried garlic, minced
- 2 tbsp chilli powder
- 1 green bell pepper, cut into strips

Directions:

1. Lightly coat the slow cooker. Add the pepper and onion in the cooker. Top with the beef. Season it with oregano, salt, chilli powder and garlic.

2. Stir in the lime juice then add the broth.

3. Cook for 8-10 hours at low heat.

4. Remove the beef from the cooking. Shred it using 2 forks then transfer to the cooker. Stir to combine.

5. Serve.

Recipe #81 - Spinach Tomato Tortellini

Ingredients:

- ¼ cup grated Parmesan cheese

- ¾ cup milk

- 1 tsp minced garlic

- ¼ tsp pepper

- 1 cup fresh spinach, chopped

- 16 oz packed cheese tortellini

- ¾ cup heavy cream

- 2 tbsp all purpose flour

- 1 ½ tsp dried basil

- ½ tsp salt

- 14.5 can tomatoes with onion and garlic, diced

Directions:

1. Pour water into a pot and bring to a boil. Add the tortellini and cook for 10 minutes or until it is tender. Prepare the remaining ingredients while you wait for the water to boil.

2. Combine the spinach, garlic, basil, salt, pepper, and tomatoes in a large pan. Place it over medium heat. Cook until the mixture starts to boil.

3. Whisk the cream, flour and milk in a bowl. Add the mixture to the saucepan along with the Parmesan cheese. Heat it through then reduce the heat. Simmer for 2 minutes or until the mixture is thick.

4. Drain the tortellini. Pour it in a saucepan with the sauce. Toss to coat and let the ingredients combine.

Recipe #82 - Pot Roast with Vegetables

Ingredients:

- 5-lb. beef chuck roast, one whole prime boneless meat, tied
- 2 cups red wine, good quality like Burgundy
- 2 cups carrots, chopped
- 2 leeks, white and light green parts, chopped
- 2 cups yellow onions, chopped
- 2 branches fresh rosemary
- 2 cups celery, chopped
- 1 can whole plum tomatoes in puree
- almond flour
- 5 garlic cloves, large, peeled and mashed
- 1 cup chicken stock, better if homemade
- 3 branches fresh thyme
- 1 chicken bouillon cube
- 1 tbsp. unsalted butter, set in room temperature
- Olive oil
- Kosher salt and pepper

Directions:

1. Preheat oven (325 degrees Fahrenheit). Dry meat by patting
   with paper towels. Season with 1 1/2 teaspoons freshly

ground pepper and a tablespoon of salt. Dredge the entire meat in flour and coat every part include the ends.

2. Sear the roast in a Dutch oven with heated 2 tablespoons of oil on medium heat. Brown for 5 minutes or until it has a good brown color. Remove roast from the pot and transfer to a large plate.

3. Combine leeks, onions, celery and garlic in the same Dutch oven. Season with the same amount of salt and pepper used for the meat above. Stir and cook for 15 minutes over medium heat. Stir occasionally to cook evenly until tender without browning. Add brandy and wine then bring the mixture to a boil.

4. Pour chicken stock and tomatoes. Drop bouillon cube and season again with small amount of salt and pepper. Secure herb branches by tying them together with a kitchen string and place inside the pot. Transfer the roast back in the pot. Bring to a boil.

5. Cover and roast for 2 1/2 hours or until meat reaches 160 degrees Fahrenheit and tender. Reduce heat to 250 degrees Fahrenheit after 60 minutes and let it simmer in its sauce.

6. Take out meat and place on a cutting board. Scoop out as much fat from the sauce and discard herb bundle. Combine veggies and 50 percent of the sauce in food processor to puree until smooth.

7. Pour the mixture back in the pot and set stove to low heat. Add the remaining sauce and simmer. Combine butter and 2 tablespoons of flour in a small bowl. Mash with a fork until completely blended. Pour it into the sauce and simmer for several minutes until it thickens.

8. Adjust taste by adding more seasoning if needed.

9. Untie roast and carve the meat. Serve by placing meat on a plate then top with a spoonful of sauce.

Recipe #83 - Tuna Salad with Pickles

Ingredients:

- 1 pinch garlic powder

- 1 tbsp dried parsley

- 1/8 tsp minced onion flakes, dried

- 1 tbsp Parmesan cheese

- 1 can white tuna, drained

- 1 tsp dried dill weed

- ¼ tsp curry powder

- 3 tbsp sweet pickle relish

- 6 tbsp mayonnaise or salad dressing

Directions:

1. Combine the tuna and mayonnaise in a bowl. Add the onion and Parmesan.

2. Season it with parsley, garlic powder, curry powder and dill. Stir well to combine. Serve it with crackers or sandwich.

Recipe #84 - Pan-Roasted Broccoli

Ingredients:

- 1 1/4 lbs. broccoli, shredded into florets and stems

- 3 tbsps. water

- 2 tbsps. vegetable oil

- Salt and pepper

Directions:

1. Heat oil in a large pan.

2. Spread and arrange broccoli stems in an even layer.

3. Let the broccoli cook without stirring for 2 minutes.

4. Add florets then toss to combine. Let it cook again for 2 minutes without stirring.

5. Pour over the water and spice mixture. Cover the pan and cook for another 2 minutes.

6. Remove cover and continue cooking until desired texture is attained.

Recipe #85 - Sesame Seared Tuna

Ingredients:

- 1 tbsp olive oil

- ½ cup sesame seeds

- 1 tbsp rice wine vinegar

- 1 tbsp honey

- ¼ cup soy sauce

- Wasabi paste

- 4 6 oz tuna steaks

- 2 tbsp sesame oil

- 1 tbsp mirin

Directions:

1. Combine the mirin, honey, sesame oil and soy sauce in a bowl. Divide it into two.

2. Add the rice vinegar to one part. This will be added to the dipping sauce.

3. Spread the sesame seeds in a plate. Coat the tuna steaks with the soy mixture. Roll it in the sesame seeds. Press it down firmly to coat.

4. Pour oil in a pan. Place it over medium heat. Sear the steaks in the pan once the oil is hot. Cook for about 30 seconds one each side.

5. Serve with the wasabi and dipping sauce.

Recipe #86 - Tuna Fry

Ingredients

- Olive oil for sautéing
- ¼ tsp black pepper, freshly ground
- 1 tsp freshly squeezed lemon juice
- 2 tsp Dijon mustard
- 7 oz albacore tuna, drained and shredded
- ¾ cup panko breadcrumbs, divided
- ½ tsp kosher salt
- 2 large eggs, beaten
- 2 green onions, chopped fine

Directions:

1. Combine the eggs, mustard, salt, pepper, lemon juice, onion, tuna and ¼ cup bread crumbs in a large mixing bowl. Stir the mixture until well combined.

2. Divide mixture into 8 rounds. Place it on a baking sheet lined with parchment paper. Set it aside and let it rest for 15 minutes.

3. Place the remaining bread crumbs into a pie plate. Coat the round with panko on all sides.

4. Pour enough oil in a large pan and place over medium heat. Add the croquettes and cook for 2-3 minutes until sides are all golden brown.

5. Remove from the cooling rack and place on top of paper towels. Let it cool for a few minutes before serving.

Recipe #87 - Buffalo Strips

Ingredients:

- 5 pieces of chicken breasts
- 8 tablespoons of almond flour
- 5 tablespoons of hot sauce
- 2 ½ tablespoons of olive oil
- Half a stick of butter
- 3 tablespoons of blue cheese
- 2 eggs
- Paprika
- Chili powder
- Salt
- Pepper
- Garlic powder
- Onion Powder

Directions:

1. Preheat oven to 205C.

2. Combine seasonings in a ramekin. Pound each chicken breast to half inch thick. Cut in half.

3. Season each side of the chicken breast. Save about 1/3 of the seasoning. Combine the remaining spice mixture with the almond flour.

4. In another bowl, crack and beat the eggs. Coat each chicken breast in the almond flour and then dip in the eggs.

5. Place chicken breasts on a cooling rack. Lay rack on top of a baking sheet. Bake chicken breast for about 15 minutes or until done.

6. After baking, broil the chicken for 5 minutes on each side. Drizzle each chicken breast with some olive oil. In a pan, mix together half a cup of hot sauce and half a stick of butter. Allow sauce to thicken.

7. Slather sauce over each chicken breast and garnish with some blue cheese.

Recipe #88 – Tomato Avocado and Olives Salad

Ingredients:

- 400 grams tomatoes

- 1 cup fresh basil leaves

- 1/4 cup olive oil

- 1/2 cup parsley leaves

- 2 avocados

- 1/4 cup red wine vinegar

- 1/2 red onion

- 1 cup Olives (black and green)

- 180 grams feta cheese

- 1 cucumber

- 1/2 ciabatta loaf

Directions:

1. Preheat the griller to high.

2. In a medium-sized bowl, combine torn basil leaves, feta cheese, pitted black olives, sliced and pitted green olives, avocado slices, red onions and thickly sliced cucumbers and tomatoes.

3. In a baking tray, add a teaspoon of extra virgin olive oil and add all the ingredients from the bowl; season them with pepper and salt.

4. Add ciabatta bread and slice them into 2.5 cubed chunks then toss it with the salad; drizzle vinegar dressing and oil.

5. Cook on the griller for about 8 minutes until the ciabatta turns golden brown and vegetables soften.

6. Serve the Tomato, Avocado, and Feta Panzanella Salad on a plate and garnish with parsley.

Recipe #89 - Chicken Salad with Fruits and Nuts

Ingredients:

- 1 package cream cheese
- 1 cup mayonnaise
- 2 teaspoons curry powder
- 1 teaspoon salt
- 6 cups cooked chicken
- 1 can pineapple
- 2/3 cup dried cranberries
- 1 cup salted almonds

Directions:

1. In a large bowl, add the cream cheese, salt and curry powder.

2. Whisk the ingredients until the cheese is fully coated by curry, and then mix the pineapple, cranberries and chicken.

3. Transfer the mixture on a plastic covered round cake pan and refrigerate overnight.

4. The following day, remove the plastic cover and invert the cake pan on a plate.

5. Toss the Creamy Chicken Salad and garnish with chopped almonds and cranberries on top.

6. Serve on a plate and enjoy your meal!

Recipe #90 - Ground Turkey with Hominy

Ingredients:

- 1 ½ pound ground turkey
- 2 cans hominy, rinsed and drained
- 2 cans un-drained diced tomatoes
- 1 chopped onion
- 1 teaspoon minced garlic
- 1 tablespoon chili powder
- 1 ½ teaspoons ground cumin
- ½ teaspoon ground mustard
- ½ teaspoon dried thyme
- ¼ teaspoon ground allspice
- ¼ teaspoon ground cinnamon
- 2 tablespoons olive oil
- Salt and pepper

Directions:

1. Heat oil in a skillet and cook turkey until meat is no longer pink.

2. Add garlic and cook for 1 minute.

3. Stir in seasonings and tomatoes.

4. Add hominy and cook for a few more minutes.

Recipe #91 - Lamb Tagine

Ingredients:

- 2 pounds lamb meat, cubed
- ¼ teaspoon ground turmeric
- ¼ teaspoon cayenne pepper
- ¼ teaspoon ground cloves
- 1 teaspoon kosher salt
- 1 pinch saffron
- ¾ teaspoon ground coriander
- 5 peeled carrots, cut into small strips
- 3 minced cloves of garlic
- 3 tablespoons olive oil
- 2 teaspoons paprika
- ½ teaspoons ground cumin
- 1 teaspoon ground cinnamon
- ½ teaspoon ground cardamom
- 1.2 teaspoon ginger
- ¾ teaspoon garlic powder
- 2 medium onions, cubed
- 1 tablespoon ginger, grated
- 1 zested lemon
- 1 tablespoon tomato paste

- 1 tablespoon cornstarch

- 1 tablespoon honey

- Water

- 1 can chicken broth

Directions:

1. Prepare a marinade bag for the lamb by combining the turmeric, paprika, cumin, cinnamon, cayenne, cardamom, cloves, ginger, salt, saffron, garlic powder and coriander in a zip lock bag. Make sure these spices are all mixed together within the bag. Toss the lamb in a bowl of olive oil before placing in the resealable bag. Keep the refrigerator overnight or for at least eight hours.

2. When ready to cook, do it in sections. The lamb should be cooked in thirds before serving. Heat some olive oil in a pan over a medium flame then throw in the lamb. Cook the lamb until it turns brown. Remove from pot and set aside.

3. Cook the onions and carrots to the pot. Cook them for five minutes. Throw in the garlic and ginger after these have cooked and stir.

4. Throw the lamb back into the pot and cook along with the chicken broth, lemon zest, honey and tomato paste. Increase heat and cook until it boils. Reduce to low heat and allow to cook for about 22 hours. Be sure to stir while cooking.

Recipe #92 - Parmesan Chicken Salad

Ingredients:

- 4 to 6 chicken breasts, boneless and skinless
- 1/2 cup Parmesan cheese, freshly grated, set extra cheese for serving
- 1 cup all-purpose flour
- 2 eggs, extra large
- 1 1/4 cups dry bread crumbs, seasoned
- 1 tbsp. water
- Kosher salt and black pepper
- Olive oil, good quality
- Unsalted butter
- Salad greens, rinsed and spun dry

Lemon Vinaigrette:

- 1/2 cup olive oil, good quality
- 1/4 cup lemon juice, freshly squeezed
- Salt and black pepper

Directions:

1. Pound chicken to quarter-inch thick using a rolling pin or meat mallet.

2. Put flour on a dinner plate and season with salt and pepper. Mix to combine well.

3. Beat eggs and add a tablespoon of water. Transfer into a shallow plate for dipping.

4. Combine parmesan cheese, and bread crumbs in another platter.

5. Coat both sides of chicken with flour first. Then dip in egg-water mixture.

6. Dredge both sides with cheese-crumbs mixture. Press lightly for crust ingredients to stick well in meat.

7. Combine a tablespoon each of olive oil and butter in a large pan. Cook chicken in batches over medium heat for 2 to 3 minutes per side. Add more shortening if needed.

8. While cooking the chicken, make lemon vinaigrette by combining juice and olive oil.

9. Season with desired amount of salt and freshly ground black pepper. Whisk to blend well.

10. Prepare greens in a bowl then toss with vinaigrette. Plate cooked chicken in a serving dish then top with greens.

11. Sprinkle with extra parmesan cheese.

Recipe #93 - Tortellini Casserole

Ingredients

- ¼ cup cilantro

- ½ cup sliced black olives

- ½ tsp sugar

- 1 ½ cups low-fat sour cream

- 15 oz can tomatoes, diced

- 9-10 oz refrigerated cheese tortellini

- ¾ cup green onions, chopped

- 2 cups Monterey Jack cheese, shredded

- ¼ cup fresh lime juice

- ½ tsp cumin

- 4 oz can green chillies, diced

Directions:

1. Set the oven at 350 degrees. Grease a 1 ½ quart casserole dish.

2. Combine the green chillies, tomatoes, tortellini and cumin in a bowl. Stir well to combine then pour in the casserole dish.

3. Combine the sour cream, sugar and lime juice in a separate bowl. Spread the mixture on top of the casserole dish. Make sure to spread it evenly.

4. Sprinkle it with cheese, green onions and olives. Top it with cilantro.

5. Cover the dish with foil and bake for 30 minutes at 350 degrees.

6. Remove the foil and bake for another 20-30 minutes until the top cheese is bubbly and golden brown.

7. Let it cool for 10 minutes. Sprinkle the cilantro on top before serving.

CHAPTER 5 DESSERTS AND SNACKS RECIPES

Recipe #94 - Curry Peanuts

Ingredients:

- 1 cup unsalted peanuts

- 1 Tbsp. freshly squeezed lime juice

- 1 Tbsp. curry powder

- Cayenne pepper, to taste

Directions:

1. Set the oven to 250 degrees F to preheat.

2. In a bowl, combine the lime juice, curry powder, and a pinch of cayenne pepper. Mix well, then add the peanuts and toss well to coat.

3. Spread the coated peanuts in a large baking sheet, then bake for 30 minutes or until browned.

4. Transfer the tray to a cooling rack and allow to cool slightly. Store in an airtight container for up to 1 week at room temperature.

Recipe #95 - Vanilla Cupcake

Ingredients:

- 2 large eggs
- 3 teaspoons baking powder
- 1 and 1/2 cups stevia
- 1 and 1/2 teaspoon vanilla
- 1/2 teaspoon salt
- 4 egg whites
- 1/2 cup shortening
- 1 cup almond milk
- 2 cups almond flour

Directions:

1. Preheat your oven to a temperature of 350 degrees F.
2. Line the muffin tins or cupcake pans with paper case liners.
3. In a large bowl, combine baking powder, salt, milk, shortening, vanilla and flour.
4. Once combined, add egg whites and use an electric mixer at high speed for 2 minutes.
5. Pour the batter into the pre-lined cupcake pans and bake in the oven for about 25 minutes.
6. Do not remove the cupcakes from the pans; let it rest for 10 minutes.
7. Transfer the cupcakes to a wire rack to cool completely.
8. Serve the classic vanilla cupcakes as it is or add candy sprinkles on top.

Recipe #96 - Sesame Hummus

Ingredients:

- 2 large garlic cloves, peeled and minced

- 2 cups canned garbanzo beans, rinsed and drained thoroughly

- ¾ cup toasted sesame seeds

- ¼ cup freshly squeezed lemon juice

- 3 Tbsp. extra virgin olive oil

- ¼ tsp. crushed red chili peppers

Directions:

1. Set the oven to 350 degrees F to preheat.

2. Spread the sesame seeds in a baking sheet and bake for 8 minutes, or until toasted.

3. Pour the toasted sesame seeds into a food processor, cover, and process until pureed.

4. Add the chili peppers, garbanzo beans, lemon juice, and garlic into the food processor and process everything until chunky smooth.

5. Spoon the mixture into a clean container, then cover and refrigerate for at least 1 hour before serving. Best served with vegetable sticks. Refrigerate for up to 1 week.

Recipe #97 - Peanut Butter Cupcake

Ingredients:

- 1 teaspoon vanilla
- 1/2 cup creamy peanut butter
- 1/8 teaspoon baking soda
- 3 and 1/2 teaspoon baking powder
- 1/2 cups stevia
- 3 large eggs
- 2 and 1/4 cups almond flour
- 1/4 cups almond milk
- 3 tablespoons baking cocoa powder
- 1 teaspoon salt

Directions:

1. Preheat your oven to a temperature of 350 degrees F.
2. Line the cupcake pans with paper liners or butter spray.
3. In a large bowl, combine all the ingredients in the list at low speed for about 30 seconds.
4. Once done, scrape the bowl to gather the batter in one place and set to a high speed for 3 minutes.
5. Fill the cupcake pans and bake in the oven for 25 minutes.
6. Do not remove the cupcakes immediately from the pans; allow it to set for 10 minutes.
7. After ten minutes, let the cupcakes cool on wire racks.
8. Serve the Choco-peanut butter cupcakes with a drizzle of chocolate syrup or a dollop of crunchy peanut butter.

Recipe #98 - Onion Garlic Yogurt Dip

Ingredients:

- 1 large garlic clove, peeled and minced

- 1 small yellow onion, peeled and diced

- ½ cup non fat plain Greek yogurt

- ¼ cup freshly grated cucumber

- 1 Tbsp. freshly squeezed lemon juice

- ½ Tbsp. minced fresh mint

- ½ Tbsp. minced fresh dill

- ½ tsp. minced fresh oregano

- 1 tsp. raw honey

- ½ tsp. extra virgin olive oil

Directions:

1. Place the yogurt in a dipping bowl then stir in the onion, lemon juice, dill, mint, oregano, honey, garlic, and olive oil. Stir well to combine.

2. Press the grated cucumber with paper towels until mostly dry. Then, stir into the yogurt mixture until evenly combined.

3. Cover the bowl and refrigerate from 1 hour to 2 days to let the flavors meld. Best served chilled with vegetable sticks.

Recipe #99 - Bran Cheesecake

Ingredients:

- 1 cup keto-friendly oat bran

- Half a stick of butter

- 2 bars cream cheese

- Half a cup of sour cream

- 2 eggs

- ½ a teaspoon of stevia powder for sweetener

- ½ teaspoon vanilla

Directions:

1. Preheat oven to 350 degrees.

2. Melt butter in a bowl.

3. Add the oat bran into the bowl of melted butter and mix.

4. Press the butter and the oat bran mixture into the bottom of a 9 inch pie plate. Make sure to cover at least half way through the sides of the pie plate.

5. Whisk together the sour cream, cream cheese, egg, dried stevia powder and vanilla. Make sure not to overbeat the filling. The texture would be a bit lumpy but rest assured that this will not affect the taste of the cheesecake.

6. Pour cheesecake mixture into the crust but make sure to leave a thin edge of the crust visible. Bake the cheesecake for 35 minutes.

7. Cool the dish on a cooling rack. Refrigerate once cooled completely. Serve.

Recipe #100 - Keto Biscuits

Ingredients:

- 18g of macadamia nut butter

- 4.5g cheddar cheese

- 3g egg whites

- Salt to taste

Directions:

1. Combine all ingredients together. Spoon mixture and drop dime size big onto a silicone lined baking sheet.

2. Bake for about 7-10minutes in a 350F oven or until the crackers turn lightly brown around the edges.

3. Once baked, allow to cool in a trivet.

Recipe #101 - Banana Milk Muffins – eat in moderation

Ingredients:

- 1 ½ cups of mashed banana

- 2 tablespoons ground of almonds

- 2 tablespoons of skimmed milk powder

- 1 whole egg, beaten

- 1/8 teaspoon of carbohydrate free baking powder

- ½ teaspoon of sweetener

- Whipped cream

Directions:

1. Pre heat oven to 190 degrees.

2. In a bowl, combine skimmed milk, ground almonds and mashed banana together.

3. Add eggs, sweetener and low carbohydrate baking powder into the mixture and combine thoroughly.

4. Divide mixture into two cupcake molds and bake for about 15 to 20 minutes.

5. Serve muffins with some whipped cream.

Recipe #102 - Fruit and Nuts Parfait

Ingredients:

- 1/3 cup full fat coconut milk

- ¼ teaspoon vanilla bean powder

- 1 tablespoon crushed raw pecans

- 2 tablespoon walnuts

- 3 tablespoons of blackberries (or any fruit that you want)

- Alcohol free stevia

Directions:

1. Place coconut milk into a bowl. Add the vanilla bean powder and mix.

2. Add stevia according to your preference.

3. Whip until fluffy.

4. Garnish with your choice of fruit, walnuts and crushed pecans.

5. Serve and enjoy.

Recipe #103 - Spicy Trail Mix

Ingredients:

- 1½ Tbsp. melted coconut oil
- 1 Tbsp. coconut sugar, add more if desired
- 1 Tbsp. pure maple syrup
- 1 tsp. cinnamon powder
- 1 tsp. sweet paprika powder
- ¼ tsp. flaky rock or kosher salt
- 1/16 tsp. cayenne pepper powder
- ½ cup raw cashew nuts
- ½ cup raw pecans
- ½ cup raw walnuts
- ½ cup raw shelled pistachio nuts

Directions:

1. Preheat oven to 175°C or 350°F. Line a rimmed cookie sheet with aluminum foil.
2. Combine all ingredients into a bowl. Spread on prepared cookie sheet in a single layer.
3. Bake for 12 to 15 minutes. Stir nuts once midway through.
4. Cool completely to room temperature before serving or storing into containers.
5. Place into single-serve resealable bags or glass jars. Label accordingly.

Recipe #104 - Choco Brownies

Ingredients:

- 1 1/4 cups almond flour
- 2/3 cup stevia or coconut sugar
- 4 1/2 Tbsp cocoa powder
- 3/4 tsp baking powder
- 2/3 tsp salt
- 6 Tbsp melted butter, cooled
- 5 eggs
- 1 1/2 tsp pure vanilla extract
- 2/3 cup 90 percent or pure dark chocolate, chopped

Directions:

1. Preheat your oven to 350 degrees F.

2. Mix the flour, cocoa powder, stevia or coconut sugar, salt, and baking powder in a mixing bowl.

3. In a separate bowl, beat together the eggs, vanilla, and melted butter.

4. Mix the egg mixture into the flour mixture very well, then stir in the chopped dark chocolate.

5. Pour the mixture into a baking pan and bake for 30 to 40 minutes. To check, poke the center with a toothpick, and if it comes out clean then it is ready.

6. Set on a cooling rack for 7 minutes, then slice into 12 pieces and serve.

Recipe #105 - Refrigerator Fudge

Ingredients:

- 1/2 cup coconut oil, softened

- 1/8 cup organic cocoa powder

- 1/8 cup coconut milk, full fat

- 1/8 cup stevia

- 1/4 tsp almond oil extract

- 1/2 tsp vanilla extract

- 1/4 tsp sea salt

Directions:

1. In a large bowl, combine the coconut oil and milk together using a hand mixer. Beat until smooth.

2. Add the rest of the ingredients into the bowl and beat until everything is combined and smooth. Adjust flavours, if desired.

3. Line a small baking pan with wax or parchment paper, making sure that the edges of the paper stand out of the pan. Pour the batter into it. Freeze for 10 minutes to make firm.

4. Take out the fudge out of the pan by pulling at the edges of the paper, and place the fudge on a cutting board.

5. With a sharp knife, slice the fudge into six servings and serve, or store in a tightly lidded container and freeze.

Recipe #106 - Zucchini Fries

Ingredients:

- ¾ cup of grated cheddar cheese
- 1/2 cup of pork rinds
- 2 egg whites
- 5 cups of zucchini sticks
- 1 tablespoon of all purpose cream

Directions:

1. Preheat the oven to 350 degree Fahrenheit.
2. Place the pork rinds in the food processor and process for about two minutes.
3. Combine the egg whites, cream, and pork rind in a bowl.
4. Dip the zucchini sticks in the pork rind mixture.
5. Place the coated zucchini sticks on a baking sheet.
6. Bake for twenty five to thirty minutes.
7. Place one cup of zucchini fries in each each container. Refrigerate the fries and heat them in a microwave oven before serving.

Recipe #107 - Microwave Tiramisu

Ingredients:

- 2 Tbsp erythritol

- 2 Tbsp unsalted butter, softened

- 1/3 cup almond flour

- 4 Tbsp vanilla whey protein powder

- 1/2 tsp baking powder

- 2 Tbsp almond milk

- 2 eggs, beaten

- 2 Tbsp instant coffee

- 4 Tbsp warm water

- 4 oz cream cheese

- 4 Tbsp heavy cream

- 2 tsp grated unsweetened chocolate

- 2 tsp unsweetened cocoa powder

Directions:

1. In a bowl, combine the erythritol and butter, then mix in the almond flour, protein powder, baking powder, almond milk, and beaten eggs.

2. Pour the mixture into 4 ramekins, then set aside for a minute.

3. Place the ramekins into the microwave and microwave for 1 minute.

4. Combine the instant coffee and water in a bowl. Mix well.

5. Place the cream cheese in a microwaveable bowl.

6. Take the cakes out of the microwave, then place the bowl of cream cheese inside and microwave for 30 seconds.

7. Slice the cakes in half, then dip the lower halves into the coffee mixture. Place the coffee dipped halves on top of the undipped halves in the ramekins.

8. Take the cream cheese out of the microwave and stir in the heavy cream. Spoon the mixture on top of the cakes and top with chocolate and cocoa powder. Serve at once, or chilled.

Recipe #108 - Red Velvet Cupcakes

Ingredients:

- 1 and ½ cups of Caster sugar
- 1 cup buttermilk
- 250g cream cheese
- 1 teaspoon baking powder
- 3 teaspoons red food coloring
- 2 tablespoons cocoa powder
- 2 and 1/3 cups of almond flour
- 100g butter
- 1 teaspoon bicarbonate of soda
- 2 eggs
- 1 teaspoon vanilla extract
- 2 teaspoons white vinegar
- ¾ cup vegetable oil
- Sprinkles (for frosting decoration)

Directions

1. Preheat your oven to 350 degrees F.
2. Line the muffin pans with paper case cups and them set aside.
3. In a large bowl, add the sifted flour, bicarbonate soda, cocoa powder, sugar and baking powder.
4. Once the dry ingredients are fully combined, add the oil, eggs, vinegar, buttermilk and food coloring.

5. Pour the batter into the muffin pans and bake in the oven for 25 minutes.

6. Cool on wire racks after the muffins cupcakes have turned light brown.

7. Prepare the cream cheese frosting while waiting for the cupcakes to set.

8. In a bowl, combine the cream cheese butter, and vanilla until smooth.

9. Transfer the mixture into icing bags and pipe over the cupcakes.

10. Dust the frosting with sprinkles and serve right away or refrigerate the cupcakes.

Recipe #109 - Vegan Nacho Cheese Dip

Ingredients:

- 2 cups cashews, raw

- 1/2 cup nutritional yeast

- 3 1/2 cup water

- 1 tsp. each of onion powder and garlic powder, heaping

- 3/4 tsp. paprika

- One 7-oz. can pimientos, undrained

- Extracted juice from two lemons

- 3 tsps. salt

Directions

1. Soak cashews for several hours to create smoother and less grainy sauce.

2. Put all the ingredients in a blender. Season with 3 teaspoons salt. pour 2 1/2 cups of water. Blend until mixed and smooth.

3. Transfer the mixture into a saucepan. Heat for 20 minutes. Stir continuously to prevent scorching.

4. Pour additional water if necessary to attain desired consistency.

5. Prepare with nachos or chips.

Recipe #110 - Nacho Hotdogs with Salsa and Guacamole

Ingredients:

For the guacamole:

- Freshly ground black pepper

- 1 jalapeno, large, diced finely

- 2 ripe Hass avocadoes, peeled, pit removed and chopped coasely

- 3 tbsps. fresh cilantro leaves, chopped

- 3 tbsps. red onion, diced finely

- 2 tbsps. canola oil

- Juice from one lime

- Salt and pepper

For Salsa:

- 4 tbsps. canola oil

- 3 tbsps. red onion, diced finely

- 3 tbsps. red wine vinegar

- 4 plum tomatoes

- 2 tsps. chipotle in adobo puree

- Salt and black pepper

For Hotdogs:

- 8 keto-friendly hotdog buns, sliced 3/4 through the bread

- 8 hotdogs, choose from chicken, beef or turkey

- 8 pickled jalapenos, sliced thinly

- 1 1/2 cups white cheddar, grated

- Fresh corn tortilla chips, crumbled coarsely

Directions:

1. Prepare guacamole by combining ingredients together in a bowl. mix well. Season with freshly ground black pepper and salt. Set aside.

2. Set grill on high heat. Brush canola oil on plum tomatoes. Season with pepper and salt.

3. Place oil-coated tomatoes on the grill. Grill until all sides are charred.

4. Remove tomatoes from the grill and sliced into half. Scrape seeds out and chop tomatoes coarsely.

5. Mix 2 tablespoons of oil, onion, chipotle puree, and vinegar in a medium-sized bowl.

6. Stir in tomatoes to the vinegar mixture. Stir well and season with pepper and salt. Set aside.

7. Preheat grill to high setting. Grill hotdogs until cooked and all sides are browned. Transfer to a plate.

8. Grill buns with the sliced part facing down. Grill for several seconds to heat and brown. Place hotdogs inside the bun.

9. Top with cheese, salsa, jalapeno, guacamole and tortilla chips. Serve.

Recipe #111 - Strawberry Cheesecake

Ingredients:

- 20 strawberries

- 1 1/2 cups almond flour

- 1 1/2 cups pecans, crushed

- 5 Tbsp Splenda

- 1/2 cup butter

- 3 lb cream cheese

- 8 eggs

- 1 Tbsp vanilla extract

- 1 Tbsp lemon juice

- 1/2 cup sour cream

Directions:

1. Preheat the oven to 400 degrees F. Grease two springform pans.
2. Place a saucepan over low flame and melt the butter. Stir in the pecans, flour, and 4 tablespoons of Splenda. Stir until thoroughly combined.
3. Divide the batter between the springform pans. Bake for 7 minutes, or until browned. Set on a wire rack to cool. Reduce oven temperature to 250 degrees F.
4. In a bowl, combine the cream cheese, eggs, 1 tablespoon of Splenda, vanilla extract, lemon juice, and sour cream.
5. Take the cheesecake base out of the oven and fill it with the cream cheese filling. Arrange the strawberries on top.
6. Bake the cheesecakes for 1 hour or until set. Serve at once or chilled.

Recipe #112- Peanut Butter Bites

Ingredients:

- 1 1/4 cups coconut oil

- 1/3 cup all natural peanut butter, sugar free

- 1/3 cup cocoa powder

- 1/4 cup liquid Splenda

Directions:

1. Place a saucepan over medium flame and heat the coconut oil. Once melted, divide between two bowls.

2. Stir the peanut butter and a third of the liquid Splenda into one bowl and mix well.

3. In the second bowl, mix in the cocoa powder and a third of the liquid Splenda. Mix well.

4. Take out 18 mini muffin cups. Divide the chocolate mixture into each cup, followed by the peanut butter mixture. Refrigerate for 6 hours or until firm.

5. Take the bites out of the refrigerator and pour the remaining liquid Splenda over each. Chill for at least 1 hour, then serve.

Recipe #113 - Colorful Cake

Ingredients:

- 1 pack yellow cake mix

- 1 16oz can vanilla frosting, less sugar

- 2 small orange gumdrops

- 2 small purple gumdrops

- 1 small red gumdrop

- 2 pretzel sticks

- 2 ½ cups coconut flakes, halved

- liquid food coloring (green, red and yellow)

Directions:

1. Follow the instructions in the package for the cake batter. Preheat oven at 350°F.

2. Grease an 8oz custard cup and a 10-inch fluted tube pan. Fill the greased custard cup with cake batter until ¾ full. Put the remaining batter on the greased 10-inch fluted tube pan.

3. Bake the custard cup for 20 to 25 minutes and the tube pan for 40 to 45 minutes or until toothpick comes out when inserted into the cake. Cool.

4. Half the tube cake crosswise and assemble the caterpillar. Put half of the tube cake in a 15x10 inches covered board. Place the other half next to first one to form a letter "s". Level top and bottom of small cake using a serrated knife. Place on whichever end to make the head.

5. Frost the head with vanilla frosting. Press about ¼ cup coconut flakes gently into the frosting. Use the purple

gumdrops for the eyes. For the mouth, place the red gumdrop in between waxed paper and flatten using rolling pin. Press the orange gumdrops on the pretzels and use as antennae.

6. Prepare three small resealable bags. Fill each bag with ¾ cup coconut flakes. For the orange color, tint one bag with red and yellow food coloring. Tint the other bag yellow and the remaining one green.

7. Frost the rest of the cake with the remaining vanilla frosting. Gently press colored coconut flakes alternately into the frosting.

Recipe #114 - Layered Mocha Cake

Ingredients:

Batter

- 1 pack regular-sized chocolate cake mix
- 3 eggs
- 1 1/3 cups brewed coffee, room temperature
- ½ cup canola oil
- ½ cup chocolate chips

Frosting

- ½ cup butter, softened
- 1 cup stevia
- ¾ cup powdered cocoa
- ½ cup shortening
- ½ cup chocolate chips
- ¼ teaspoon almond extract
- 7 tablespoons brewed coffee, room temperature

Directions:

1. Whisk together cake mix, oil, eggs and brewed coffee on slow speed for 30 seconds. Adjust speed to medium and whisk batter for another 2 minutes.

2. Preheat oven at 350°F. Grease and flour two 8-inch round baking pans. Then, pour batter evenly into each one.

3. Bake for 30 to 35 minutes or until toothpick/fork inserted in the middle of the cake comes out clean. Cool for 5 minutes and invert on a wire rack while still warm. Top each cake with ¼ cups chocolate chips and spread evenly when melted. Cool in the refrigerator.

4. In a large mixing bowl, cream butter and stir in shortening and confectioner's sugar. Whisk until fluffy and light. Add cocoa powder and vanilla extract. Stir in 5 tablespoons of brewed coffee, one tablespoon at a time. Beat with electric mixer set on low until fluffy and creamy.

5. Spread frosting between layers and all over the cake.

6. In a microwaveable bowl, combine remaining coffee and chocolate chips. Melt in the microwave for about a minute in medium high setting. Mix until mixture is smooth.

7. Gently drizzle on top of the cake, allowing some to drip on the sides.

Recipe #115 - Tiramisu Cake

Ingredients:

Batter

- 1 18.25oz pack Moist Cake Mix

- ¼ cup brewed Coffee, room temperature

- 1 tablespoon of Coffee Flavored Liquor

- 1 teaspoon Instant Coffee Powder

Filling

- 1 8oz pack Mascarpone Cheese

- 2 tablespoons of Coffee Flavored Liquor

- ½ cup stevia

Frosting

- ¼ cup stevia

- 2 tablespoons Coffee Flavored Liquor

- 2 cups Heavy Cream

Garnish

- 1 1oz square Semi-sweet Chocolate

- 2 tablespoons Cocoa Powder, unsweetened

Directions:

1. Preheat oven to 350°F. Grease and lightly flour bottom of 3, 9-inch baking pans.

2. Follow the instructions in the package for making the cake batter. Put 2/3 batter on each of the two baking pans. Mix

instant coffee into the remaining batter and pour into the last baking pan.

3. Bake for 20 to 25 minutes or until no more batter sticks to the toothpick inserted into the cake. Cool in the pan for 10 minutes. Afterwards, invert in a wire rack for further cooling.

4. In a cup, mix together brewed coffee and liquor until well blended. Set aside.

5. For the filling, combine Mascarpone cheese, confectioner's sugar and liquor in a small bowl. Set electric mixer to low and whisk until mixture is smooth and no clumps are seen. Cover with plastic wrap and let cool in the refrigerator.

6. For the frosting, mix together cream, confectioner's sugar and liquor using an electric mixer set on medium high. Mix until frosting is stiff. Divide the cream mixture. Fold the other half of the frosting into the filling. Use a large wooden spoon to make sure they incorporate well. Refrigerate both (frosting and filling).

7. Meanwhile, poke holes in the cake using a thin skewer. Make them an inch apart. Place one cake on a serving plate and pour over 1/3 of the coffee mixture on top. Put half of the filling on top of the cake and spread evenly. Place the other cake on top and poke holes on it just like the first one. Pour over what's left of the coffee mixture and spread with filling.

8. Place remaining cake on top of the other cakes and apply frosting on all sides, until the top. Using a sieve, lightly dust top of cake with powdered cocoa.

9. Use a vegetable peeler to run down the edge of the chocolate bar to make chocolate curls. Use these chocolate curls to garnish top of the cake.

10. Cool in the refrigerator for 30 minutes before serving.

Recipe #116 - Coffee Cake

Ingredients:

- 1 cup stevia
- 1 ¾ cups almond flour
- ¾ cup cocoa powder, unsweetened
- 2 teaspoons of baking soda
- 2 large eggs
- 1 teaspoon baking powder
- 1 teaspoon salt
- 1 teaspoon vanilla extract
- ½ cup vegetable oil
- 1 cup brewed coffee, room temperature
- 1 cup buttermilk

Directions:

1. Preheat oven to 350°F. Grease and flour a 9x13 inches pan or two 9-inches round cake pans.

2. Combine all dry ingredients (white sugar, baking powder, cocoa powder, flour, baking soda, and salt) in a mixing bowl. Make a well in the center and add all wet ingredients (vanilla extract, vegetable oil, brewed coffee, buttermilk and eggs). Set electric mixer to medium and beat for 2 minutes or until batter becomes thin.

3. Pour into greased cake pans and bake for 30 to 40 minutes or until toothpick comes out clean when inserted in the cake.

4. Allow to cool for 10 minutes. Remove from pan and let cool completely on wire rack. You may use any filling or frosting of your choice.

Recipe #117 - Carrot Cake

Ingredients

- 2 cups almond Flour
- 2 cups Carrots, shredded
- 1 ½ cups stevia
- 1 cup Raisins
- 1 cup Coconut Flakes
- 1 cup Walnuts, chopped
- ¾ cup Vegetable Oil
- ¾ cup Buttermilk
- 1 8oz can crushed Pineapple, juice added
- 2 teaspoons of Baking Soda
- 2 teaspoons Cinnamon, ground
- 2 teaspoons Vanilla Extract
- ¼ teaspoon Salt
- 3 Eggs

Directions

1. Preheat oven to 350°F. Grease and flour an 8x12 inch baking pan.

2. Sift together flour, salt, baking soda and ground cinnamon. Set aside.

3. Combine oil, sugar, buttermilk, vanilla and eggs in a mixing bowl. Whisk until all ingredients are well combined. Add flour mixture. Whisk until all ingredients are well combined.

4. In a separate bowl, combine carrots, walnuts, coconuts, raisins and pineapple. Add mixture into the batter and fold using a large wooden spoon or a heavy whisk.

5. Pour into the greased baking pan and bake for an hour or when toothpick comes out clean when inserted into the cake.

6. Cool for 20 minutes and serve.

Recipe #118 - Blackberry Cake

Ingredients:

Topping

- 1/3 cup almond Flour
- 1/3 cup stevia Sugar
- ½ teaspoon Cinnamon, ground
- 2 tablespoons Butter, softened

Batter

- 1 ½ cups almond Flour
- ¾ cup Plain Yogurt
- 1 cup Bran Cereal
- 1 cup Blackberries, fresh or frozen
- ½ cup stevia
- 1/3 cup Butter, softened
- 1 ½ teaspoons Baking Powder
- ½ teaspoon Baking Soda
- 1 teaspoon Vanilla
- 1 teaspoon Lemon Peel, grated
- 1 egg

Directions:

1. Preheat oven to 350°F. Crush cereal in food processor or place in a resealable plastic bag and roll with rolling pin or pound with meat mallet.

2. Grease and lightly flour 9-inch baking pan. Combine all topping ingredients in a mixing bowl and set aside.

3. In another bowl, sift together flour, crushed cereal, baking soda and baking powder. Reserve for later.

4. In a large mixing bowl, beat butter and sugar using spoon until mixture becomes fluffy. Add egg, vanilla and lemon peel. Beat with electric mixer set to low until creamy. Mix in flour mixture and beat over low until all ingredients are incorporated.

5. Gently mix blackberries into the batter using a whisker. Spread batter evenly into greased baking pan. Sprinkle with topping on top.

6. Bake for 40 to 45 minutes or until no batter sticks to inserted toothpick. Serve while still warm

Recipe #119 - Carrot Fries

Ingredients:

- 2 cups of carrot sticks
- Salt and pepper, as needed
- 2 tablespoons of chopped basil
- Parmesan cheese

Directions:

1. Preheat the oven to 400 degrees.
2. In a bowl, combine the salt, pepper, and olive oil.
3. Grease the baking pan with a little olive oil.
4. Place the carrots in the pan and bake for fifteen minutes.
5. Remove the carrots from the oven. Add the Parmesan cheese.
6. Place the fries in four small microwaveable containers. Chill in the refrigerator and heat in the microwave oven before serving.

Recipe #120 - Cheesy Pear

Ingredients

- 2 pieces of large pear
- 1 cup of skim feta cheese
- 4 tablespoons of grounded nutmeg

Directions:

1. Cut the pear into half.
2. Preheat the oven to 300 degrees Fahrenheit.
3. Combine the grounded nutmeg and the feta cheese. Set aside.
4. Place the halved pears on a baking sheet and bake for ten minutes.
5. Remove the pears from the oven and place the feta cheese on top.
6. Place the pork rinds in the food processor and process for about two minutes.
7. Place each pear in a small microwaveable container. Heat in the microwave for 30 to 60 seconds before serving.

Recipe #121 - Cinnamon and Peanut Butter Bites

Ingredients:

- 6 Tbsp unsweetened cocoa powder

- 6 Tbsp coconut oil

- 2/3 cup all natural peanut butter, sugar free

- 1/3 cup finely chopped almonds or walnuts

- 1 1/2 tsp vanilla extract

- 1/3 tsp cinnamon

- 5 Tbsp Splenda

- Sea salt

Directions:

1. Place the coconut oil into a microwaveable bowl and melt in the microwave for about 40 seconds.

2. Take out the bowl from the microwave and mix the cocoa, vanilla, and Splenda with the coconut oil. Stir until you get a smooth consistency. Stir in the chopped almonds or walnuts.

3. Pour the mixture into a baking sheet, creating an even layer.

4. In a separate bowl, combine the peanut butter and cinnamon. Mix well, then pour on top of the chocolate mixture. Sprinkle a bit of sea salt on top of the mixture.

5. Place the baking sheet in the freezer and freeze for at least half an hour. Slice into squares, then serve.

Recipe #122 - Coconut Blueberry Bites

Ingredients:

- 1/2 cup fresh or frozen blueberries

- 1/3 cup coconut oil

- 1/4 cup butter

- 2 oz cream cheese, softened

- 2 Tbsp coconut cream

- Splenda

Directions:

1. Arrange the blueberries in a small saucepan, creating a single layer. Place over low flame, then add the butter and coconut oil. Cook until butter and coconut oil are melted, then swirl everything to mix.

2. Remove the pan from the flame and set aside to cool for about 8 minutes.

3. Once cool, stir in the cream cheese and coconut cream. Mix well, then gradually add the Splenda. Sweeten to taste.

4. Transfer the mixture into a dish, then cover and freeze for at least 1 hour. Slice and serve at once.

Recipe #123 - Keto Snickerdoodles

Ingredients:

- 2 ¼ cups almond flour

- ¾ cup butter, softened

- 1 ½ cups and 3 Tbsp granulated erythritol

- 1/3 tsp baking soda

- 1/6 tsp sea salt

- 2 small eggs

- 1 ½ tsp ground cinnamon

- 1 ½ tsp vanilla extract

Directions:

1. Set the oven to 350 degrees F.

2. Combine the baking soda, salt, and almond flour in a bowl.

3. In another bowl, beat the butter and 1 ½ cups of erythritol until creamy using an electric mixer. Add the vanilla extract and eggs, then beat until smooth.

4. Gradually mix the flour mixture into the butter mixture, then set aside.

5. In a dish, combine the cinnamon and remaining erythritol.

6. Divide the dough into 18 pieces, then roll them in the erythritol and cinnamon mixture.

7. Arrange the balls on a dry baking sheet and flatten using the bottom of a cup spoon.

8. Bake for 8 minutes, or until golden brown. Set on a cooling rack for 5 minutes before serving.

Recipe #124 - Banana-Walnut Cupcakes

Ingredients:

For the Cupcake Batter

- 2 and 1/2 cups almond flour
- 1 cup stevia
- 1 teaspoon baking soda
- 3/4 cup buttermilk
- 1 teaspoon vanilla extract
- 1/2 teaspoon salt
- 2 medium ripe bananas
- 1 and 1/4 teaspoons baking powder
- 1/2 cup softened butter
- 3 large eggs

For the Nut Topping

- 1 cup chopped walnuts
- 4 tbsp stevia
- 1/4 cup heavy cream
- 1/2 cup butter

For the Cupcake Filling

- 1 tablespoon butter

- 1/2 cups stevia
- 1 large egg
- 3 tablespoons almond flour
- 1 teaspoon vanilla extract
- 1 cup 2% milk
- 2 ripe bananas
- Whipped cream
- 1/4 teaspoon salt

Directions:

1. Preheat the oven to 350 degrees F.
2. Line your cupcake pans with paper liners or grease with butter spray.

Cupcake Topping

1. In a small saucepan, heat the butter, cream and brown sugar.
2. Pour the butter mixture into the cupcake pans and add chopped walnuts.

Cupcake Batter

1. In a medium-sized bowl, mix soft butter, vanilla and mashed bananas.
2. Use a handheld mixer to combine all batter mixture with 4 eggs.

3. Add one egg for every ingredient addition to make the batter fluffy.

4. In a small bowl, mix the baking powder, baking soda, flour and salt.

5. Add the last batch of the flour and buttermilk before transferring the batter to the cupcake pans.

6. Pour the batter on top of the previously prepared walnuts and sugar layer. Bake the pans in the oven for about 20 minutes.

Cupcake Filling

1. Meanwhile, while the cupcakes are baking in the oven, prepare the ingredients in a medium-sized bowl.

2. Combine the sugar and salt to make the filling then add it in a medium saucepan; pour in the milk and continue heating.

3. When the mixture comes to a boil, remove the saucepan from the heat and add half a cup of hot mixture in a small bowl.

4. Whisk one tempered egg in the same mixture and stir in butter and vanilla.

5. Cool for 15 minutes before refrigerating for an hour.

Cupcake Presentation

1. Be creative with your cupcakes by slicing them into 3 parts.

2. Fill the first layer with the butter and vanilla filling and then banana slices and chopped walnuts for the second layer.

3. Top the cupcake with whipped cream and a dash of cinnamon.

Recipe #125 - Blackberry Pudding

Ingredients:

- 1/2 cup coconut flour
- 1/2 tsp baking powder
- 4 Tbsp coconut oil
- 4 Tbsp heavy cream
- 4 Tbsp butter
- 4 tsp lemon juice
- Zest of 2 lemons
- 10 large egg yolks
- 20 drops liquid stevia
- 4 Tbsp erythritol
- 1/2 cup blackberries

Directions:

1. Preheat the oven to 350 degrees F.
2. In a bowl, combine the coconut flour and baking powder.
3. In a separate bowl, beat the egg yolks until thoroughly combined. Whisk in the stevia and erythritol, followed by the lemon juice and zest, heavy cream, butter, and coconut oil. Mix well.
4. Sift the dry ingredients into the egg yolk mixture and mix well.

5. Divide the mixture among 4 ramekins, then distribute the blackberries evenly to each serving.

6. Bake for 25 minutes. Serve at room temperature or chilled.

CHAPTER 6 BONUS RECIPES

Irish Lamb Stew

Ingredients:

- 6 pounds lamb shoulder, boneless and cut into small pieces
- ½ teaspoon ground black pepper
- 3 cloves minced garlic
- ½ cup water
- 2 teaspoons white sugar
- 2 cut onions
- 1 teaspoon thyme, dried
- 1 cup white wine
- 1 ½ pounds bacon, diced
- ½ teaspoon salt
- ½ cup all-purpose flour
- 1 chopped onion
- 4 cups beef stock
- 4 cups diced carrot
- 3 potatoes
- 2 bay leaves

Directions:

1. Combine the lamb with the pepper, salt and flour in a mixing bowl. Make sure to toss the lamb in the other ingredients.

2. Throw the tossed lamb into a frying pan. Make sure the pan has been lined with drippings from the bacon cooked before the lamb was prepared.

3. When the lamb turns brown from cooking, remove and place into a stock pot.

4. On the previous frying pan, sauté the garlic and onion. Wait for them to become golden. Be sure to de-glaze the pan with half a cup of water.

5. Throw in the onion and garlic mixture in the pot along with the beef stock. Cover the pot and cook for about an hour and a half.

6. Throw in the rest of the ingredients into the pot, including the wine and reduce the heat. Cook for an additional twenty minutes for the vegetables to become soft and edible. Check the tenderness of the vegetables with a fork. Can be served immediately after cooking.

Sausage Casserole

Ingredients:

- 1lb sage-flavor breakfast sausage
- 6 large eggs
- 12oz mild cheddar cheese, shredded
- 3 cups potatoes, drained, shredded and pressed
- 1 16oz pack curd cottage cheese
- ¼ cup butter, melted
- ½ cup onion, shredded

Directions:

1. Preheat oven to a temperature of 375°F. Grease a 9x13 inches baking pan.
2. Heat a deep skillet over medium heat. Cook sausage until evenly brown on all sides. Drain and crumble. Reserve for later.
3. Mix butter and shredded potatoes in the greased baking dish.
4. In a mixing bowl, combine onions, cottage cheese, cheddar cheese and eggs. Spread on top of potato mixture.
5. Bake for 1 hour or until toothpick comes out clean when inserted in the casserole. Allow it to cool for about 5 minutes prior to serving.

Creamy Chicken Casserole

Ingredients:

- 3 skinless chicken breasts, deboned and halved lengthwise
- 1/3 cup all-purpose flour
- ½ cup cream sherry wine
- 1 18oz can creamy mushroom soup
- 6 slices muenster cheese
- 3 tablespoons vegetable oil
- 3 tablespoons parsley, chopped
- 2 tablespoons butter
- salt
- pepper

Directions:

1. Preheat oven to a temperature of 350°F.

2. Sprinkle chicken with salt and pepper. Place flour in a shallow plate and coat all sides of chicken. Pat off excess flour.

3. Heat oil in a skillet over medium heat. Fry chicken until both sides are brown. Place chicken in a 3 quart glass baking dish.

4. In the same skillet, melt butter over medium heat. Sautee mushrooms and season with salt and pepper. Cook until mushrooms are golden brown. Pour in sherry and cook for another minute. Add soup and mix well. Heat thoroughly.

5. Spread mushroom sauce over chicken. Top each chicken with a slice of cheese. Fold cheese slice into half if it's too wide for the chicken.

6. Cover baking dish with foil and bake for 30 minutes. Turn oven into boil setting. Remove foil from baking dish. Broil for 1 to 2 minutes or until cheese is brown. Remove from oven and cool.

7. Garnish with parsley.

Spiced Lamb Kebabs

Ingredients:

- 1 lb small zucchini, halved lengthwise and cut crosswise into 1 inch pieces
- Kosher salt and ground pepper
- 2 garlic, minced
- 1 tsp ground cumin
- ¼ cup fat-free plain Greek yogurt
- 2 lb lean leg of lamb, trimmed and cut into cubes
- 1 tbsp extra-virgin olive oil, more for brushing
- ½ tsp ground allspice
- 1 tbsp hot paprika
- Warmed pita bread, for serving

Directions:

1. Whisk the yogurt in a large bowl. Add the garlic, allspice, cumin and 1 tbsp of olive oil.
2. Season it with ½ tsp salt and ½ tsp pepper.
3. Add the lamb and stir until coated. Let it sit in room temperature for 1-3 hours.
4. Preheat the grill. Thread the zucchini and lamb into 12 long skewers. Coat it with oil and season with salt and pepper.
5. Cook in the grill over moderate heat. Turn it once and cook until the outside is browned and the inside is medium rare. Serve the lamb with pita.

Mixed Vegetable Kabobs

Ingredients:

Vegetables

- 12 pineapple chunks
- 12 slices yellow squash
- 12 small onions
- 12 slices Japanese eggplants
- 12 slices zucchini
- 2 yellow peppers, cut into squares
- 12 mushrooms
- 12 cherry tomatoes

Marinade

- ¼ cup pineapple juice
- 1 tsp fresh ginger, grated
- 1 ½ tsp ground pepper
- 1 tsp thyme
- 2 tsp salt
- 1/8 cup Worcestershire sauce
- ¼ cup light soy sauce
- 1 tbsp honey
- 2 garlic cloves, crushed
- 1 tsp oregano
- 1 tsp parsley
- 1 tbsp dry mustard
- ¾ cup olive oil

Directions:

1. Combine all of the marinade ingredients in a food blender and process it for 30 seconds.
2. Pour the marinade mixture in a zip lock bag. Place it in the refrigerator for an hour.
3. Thread the vegetables on the skewers and grill at medium heat. Make sure to brush it with the marinade until it is cooked.

Crock Pot Roast Beef (Slow Cooker) Recipe

Ingredients:

- 4 lbs. chuck roast, boneless
- 1 beef bouillon cube
- 12 French rolls, split
- 1 tsp. each of dried, thyme, dried and crushed rosemary, and garlic powder
- 1/2 cup soy sauce
- 3 to 4 peppercorns
- 1 bay leaf

Directions:

1. Place roast inside the slow cooker.

2. Mix the remaining ingredients, except for the bread, in a small bowl. Stir until completely blended. Pour mixture over meat. Add water until the meat is almost covered.

3. Cover pot and cook over low settings for 7 hours or until fork tender.

4. Take out meat, but save broth for serving later.

5. Shred meat using a fork and serve with sandwich rolls.

6. Set broth on the side, which will be used for dipping.

Six Cheeses Tortellini

Ingredients:

- 2 packs fresh cheese tortellini
- 8 oz 6-cheese Italian blend (Asiago, Romano, smoked Provolone, Mozzarella, Parmesan and Fontina)
- 1 cup whole milk
- 1/8 tsp cayenne pepper
- ¼ cup processed liquid cheese spread
- 2 tbsp. butter
- Salt

Directions:

1. Melt the butter in a saucepan. Add the milk and simmer. Stir the mixture then add the cheese gradually.
2. Stir the mixture until it completely melts and the mixture begins to bubble. Add the cayenne.
3. Cook the tortellini in a pot of boiling water for 4 minutes or until it is cooked. Drain.
4. Add the cheese sauce and toss to coat the mixture.
5. Divide the sauce and tortellini among the bowl then serve.

Salisbury Steak

Ingredients

For the gravy

- 1 tsp cornstarch
- 1 tsp seasoning sauce
- 2 cups beef broth, more if needed
- Salt and pepper
- 4 dash Worcestershire
- 1 tbsp ketchup
- 1 whole onion, halved and thinly sliced

For the meat

- 1 tbsp butter
- 1 cube beef bouillon, crumbled
- 2 tsp dry mustard
- ½ cup seasoned breadcrumbs
- 1 tbsp olive oil
- Salt and pepper
- 4 dashes Worcestershire sauce
- 1 tbsp ketchup
- 1 ½ lb lean ground beef

Directions:

1. Combine the ground beef, ketchup, Worcestershire sauce, salt, pepper, bouillon, dry mustard and bread crumbs. Knead the mixture until combined. Form it into 4-6 patties depending on your preference. Draw lines on the steak to give it a 'steak' appearance.

2. Fry the patties in a pan with oil and butter. Cook until it is no longer pink in the middle. Remove from pan and discard excess grease.

3. Make the gravy. Reduce the heat then add the sliced onion. Cook until it is golden brown for a few minutes. Add the ketchup, seasoning, beef stock and Worcestershire sauce. Add the cornstarch. Stir the mixture until it is thick. Sprinkle salt and pepper to season.

4. Return the patties to the gravy. Let it simmer for a couple minutes.

Tuna Steak

Ingredients:

- 4 4oz tuna steaks
- ½ tsp fresh oregano, chopped
- 2 tbsp fresh parsley, chopped
- 2 tbsp olive oil
- ¼ cup orange juice
- ½ tsp black pepper
- 1 garlic clove, minced
- 1 tbsp lemon juice
- ¼ cup soy sauce

Directions:

1. Combine the soy sauce, olive oil, parsley, oregano, garlic, pepper, lemon juice and orange juice in a large dish. Add the tuna steaks and let it marinade for 30 minutes.

2. Preheat the grill. Spread oil on the grill. Cook the tuna for 5 minutes on each side. Baste with the marinade. Cook until done.

Grilled Lamb Chops

Ingredients:

- 2 teaspoons salt
- 1 tablespoon garlic, minded
- 2 tablespoons olive oil
- 2 pounds lamb chops
- ¼ cup white vinegar, distilled
- ½ teaspoon black pepper
- 1 onion, sliced thinly
- 2 tablespoons olive oil

Directions:

1. Start by preparing a grill for the chops. Leave the grill on medium heat.

2. Place the lamb in a resealable bag containing a mixture of salt, pepper vinegar, onion, garlic and olive oil. Make sure to shake the bag with the chops inside so that the ingredients seep into the lamb.

3. When the lamb has been marinated in the mixture, wrap the lamb in foil. This will prevent the chops from burning when placed over the grill. Make sure there isn't any marinade dripping from the chops before wrapping in the foil. Place the foiled chops over the grill and let them site for about three minutes for each side. These can be served immediately.

Lamb Cake

Ingredients:

- 2 ½ teaspoons baking powder
- 1 ¼ cups white sugar
- 1 cup milk
- 4 egg whites
- 2 ¼ cups almond flour
- ½ teaspoon salt
- ½ cup butter
- 1 teaspoon vanilla extract

Directions:

1. Prepare the batter by creaming the butter and the sugar together in a bowl. When it turns fluffy, combine it with sifted cake flour with salt. Throw the milk into the mixture. Be sure to be stirring the batter before adding more ingredients. This will help keep the consistency of the batter. Finish by finally adding the vanilla extract. Stir until the smell of the extract is noticeable. More vanilla can be added to improve the flavour.

2. In a separate mixing bowl, beat the egg whites. When soft peaks begin to form, fold a portion of the whites into the earlier made batter. Mix for a while then throw in the remaining egg whites. This will help tighten the batter and make it easier to bake. More eggs can be added if the batter does not seem as tight as expected. Do it by folding in one egg white at a time.

3. Coat your baking mold with vegetable oil. Wipe the oil after leaving it for about five minutes. This will allow flour to stick to the mold when you prepare it for the batter. Leave the flour stuck to the mold and make sure you cover the whole inner are of the mold when you coat it iwth flour.

4. When pouring the batter into the mold, be sure to do it slowly. This can be done by stirring the bowl of batter with a spatula as it is tilted towards the opening of the cake mold. Be sure not to just dump everything into the mold. This will create a lop-sided cake. It will also result into a cake with many air pockets. Cover the mold with a locked seal.

5. Before placing the cake in a pre-heated oven, stick a toothpick into the batter. Bake the cake for about an hour. Check if the cake is done by pulling out the toothpick every now and then. If the toothpick comes out clean, then the cake is done.

6. When removing the cake from the oven, allow it to sit for about fifteen minutes. This will allow all the excess steam to come out before taking off the lid. Remove the lid slowly, allowing the steam to gush out bit by bit. Doing this suddenly might add too much stress to the cake and it may not stand upright.

7. Using a spatula, carve the cake out of the mold by moving it along the insides of the mold, being careful not to damage the cake. Taking out the cake immediately without letting it sit or carving it out with a spatula will make it a messy ordeal. A thin cake cutter can also be used to take it out. Dumping the cake upside down on a plate or bowl might also damage the cake.

8. When removed from the mold, the cake can be decorated with easy-to-prepare icing mixes. Home-made icing can be made as well. It is also optional to add sprinkles and other decorative supplements to the cake.

9. The consistency and color of the cake will resemble cooked lamb. It can be designed or cut to look like a cut of lamb as well. Including actual meat in a cake will result in a well-done cake with the taste of undercooked lamb meat.

Butter Sautéed Mushrooms

Ingredients:

- 1 lb. fresh mushrooms, sliced
- 3 green onions, retain tops, chopped
- 1/4 cup dry white wine
- 1/4 cup butter or margarine, melted
- 2 tsps. Worcestershire sauce
- 1/8 tsp. garlic powder
- Salt and pepper

Directions:

1. Heat melted butter in a pan.

2. Sauté green onions until translucent and tender.

3. Add the remaining ingredients.

4. Season with salt and pepper. Stir well.

5. Continue cooking uncovered for 30 minutes over low heat. Remove from heat once mushrooms are tender. Serve

Cream of Mushroom Soup

Ingredients:

- 8 oz. fresh mushrooms, wash cleaned and chopped
- 2 qts. stock of choice, choose from bouillon or canned vegetable, chicken or beef variant
- 2/3 cup flour
- 1 cup milk or half-and-half cream
- 6 tbsps. butter

Directions:

1. Heat butter in a small pan or saucepan. Sauté mushrooms lightly.

2. Put flour and cook for 5 minutes while stirring constantly. Pour stock slowly. Stir until all ingredients are combined.

3. Simmer for 10 minutes. Pour cream and stir until blended. Serve.

Chicken Pad Thai

Ingredients

Sauce:

- 3 tbsps. fish sauce
- 3 tbsps. rice vinegar
- Juice from one lime
- 1/4 cup stevia
- red pepper flakes, crushed, to taste

Noodles:

- 1 lb. chicken breasts, skinless and boneless, sliced into bite-size pieces
- Vegetable noodles such as zucchini
- 2 eggs, beaten
- 4 green onions, medium, sliced
- 4 tbsps. canola oil
- 3 garlic cloves, minced
- 2 tbsps. soy sauce

Garnish:

- 1/4 cup fresh cilantro, chopped
- 1/3 cup peanuts, chopped

Directions:

1. Place boiling water in a large bowl.

2. Soak noodles in water for 10 minutes until soft. Drain and set aside.

3. While soaking, combine sauce ingredients. Mix well and set aside.

4. Heat 2 tablespoons of the oil in a heavy pan over medium to high heat.

5. Sauté garlic and onions for 2 minutes.

6. Add chicken and season with soy sauce. Fry for 5 minutes or until meat is cooked. Transfer chicken to a plate and keep warm.

7. Heat the remaining oil in the same pan.

8. Cook eggs for 3 minutes until firm and scrambled.

9. Add chicken, noodles and sauce in the pan. Stir-fry for 2 minutes.

10. Add bean sprouts and cook for additional 3 minutes until sprouts and noodles are tender. Stir frequently as you cook.

11. If the mixture is too dry, pour 1/4 cup water and continue cooking.

12. Transfer to a large or individual bowls. Top with cilantro and peanuts.

Chicken and Shrimp Pad Thai

Ingredients

- 1/4 lb. Vegetable noodles such as zucchini
- 4 oz. chicken breast or thigh, skinless and boneless, sliced into strips
- 3 tbsps. canola oil
- 12 shrimp, medium to large, peeled and deveined
- 1/2 cup mixed vegetables, combination of zucchini, carrots and yellow squash, cut into julienne slices
- 1 tbsp. creamy peanut butter
- 1 tbsp. soy sauce
- 1 tbsp. cider vinegar
- 1 tbsp. water
- 1 tbsp. packed light brown sugar
- 1 tsp. each of minced ginger and garlic
- 1 tsp. Asian chili paste

Garnishing:

- Fresh cilantro leaves
- Romaine lettuce, chopped
- Lime wedges
- Peanuts, chopped

Directions

1. Combine peanut butter, soy sauce, chili paste and water. Mix well until smooth. Set aside.

2. Heat canola oil in a wok.

3. Sauté garlic and ginger for a minute until fragrant.

4. Add chicken, vegetables and shrimp. Cook until the meat and seafood are cooked and browned.

5. Add drained noodles. Toss well to coat each strand.

6. Pour the spice mixture, vinegar and brown sugar into the cooking noodles. Toss well to coat everything with sauce.

7. Arrange chopped romaine on a serving plate. Spoon the noodles over the greens and plate with the remaining garnishing.

Avocado Seafood Salsa

Ingredients:

- 2 ripe avocados (medium, peeled, pitted and chopped)
- 1 pound of small shrimp, cooked, and then peeled, deveined and chopped
- 2 tomatoes (medium), seeded and chopped
- 1 sweet red pepper (medium), chopped
- 1 cup of fresh cilantro, minced
- 3/4 cup thinly sliced green onions
- 3 tablespoons of lime juice
- 1/2 cup of chopped cucumber (seeded and peeled)
- 1 jalapeno, seeded and chopped
- 1/4 teaspoon pepper
- 1 teaspoon salt

Directions:

1. In a large bowl, combine all the ingredients.

2. You can eat this appetizing salsa by itself or with tortilla chips.

Avocado-Tomato Salad

Ingredients:

- 2 avocados (ripe), peeled, pitted and diced
- 1/2 cup of nicoise olives, pitted and roughly chopped
- 2 ripe beefsteak tomatoes (medium), diced
- 1 cup of canned chickpeas, drained, rinsed and then drained again
- 1/4 cup champagne vinegar
- 2 tablespoons of flat-leaf parsley, roughly torn
- 1/4 cup extra-virgin olive oil
- 1/2 teaspoon of smoked paprika
- 1 teaspoon of ground cumin
- Salt (to taste)
- black pepper, freshly ground(to taste)
- 2 ounces of tortilla chips, blue corn variety

Directions:

1. In a large bowl, gently toss the avocados, olives, tomatoes, parsley, chickpeas, olive oil, vinegar, paprika, cumin, salt and pepper.

2. Crumble the tortilla chips over the salad and then serve. This makes 4 servings.

Beef Kabobs

Ingredients:

- 8 metal skewers or as needed
- 1 ½ lb lean beef, cut into cubes
- 1 tsp coarsely cracked black pepper
- 1 tbsp Worcestershire sauce
- ¼ cup lemon juice
- 1/3 cup vegetable oil
- 16 mushroom caps
- 1 ½ tsp salt
- 1 garlic clove, minced
- 1 tbsp prepared mustard
- ½ cup soy sauce
- 2 green bell peppers cut into chunks
- 1 large onion, cut into squares
- 1 red bell pepper, cut into chunks

Directions:

1. Combine the soy sauce, mustard, garlic, salt, vegetable oil, lemon juice, Worcestershire sauce and black pepper in a bowl. Whisk the ingredients and pour it in a sealable bag.
2. Add the beef and turn the bag to coat it with the marinade. Let it soak for at least 8 hours.
3. Add the mushrooms to the bag. Let it marinate for another 8 hours.
4. Set the grill at high heat. Spread the oil on the grill. Remove the beef and mushrooms from marinade and shake off any excess liquid.
5. Pour the marinade in a pan and boil over medium heat. Reduce heat and simmer for 10 minutes. Set it aside.

6. Thread the green bell pepper, red bell pepper, onion, beef and mushroom into the skewers. Repeat until all of the ingredients are used.
7. Cook the kebob for 15 minutes. Turn it frequently and brush it with the marinade until it is browned on all sides and the meat is cooked through.

CHAPTER 7 31-DAY MEAL PLAN

This 31-day meal plan is a mere sample. You can substitute Keto Diet safe ingredients that are more readily available in your area. Always stick to recommended portions per meal to avoid weight gain.

Also, do not be afraid to use your favorite Keto-safe ingredients over and over. These would make this diet easier to gastronomically accept and prepare, and may save you money and time in the long run.

Day 1

Breakfast - Baked Eggs Wrapped in Bacon

Lunch - Beef Stroganoff with Mushrooms

Dinner - Sweet and Spicy Shrimp

Snack/Dessert - Curry Peanuts

Day 2

Breakfast – Avocado, Broccoli, and Bacon in a Pan

Lunch - Broccoli Soup

Dinner - Lemon- Garlic Shrimp

Snack/Dessert - Vanilla Cupcake

214

Day 3

Breakfast – Avocado Breakfast Toast

Lunch - Chicken Strips and Broccoli

Dinner - Sausage and Vegetable Soup

Snack/Dessert Sesame Hummus

Day 4

Breakfast - Spicy and Cheesy Sausage

Lunch - Cream of Asparagus Soup

Dinner – Caribbean-Style Chicken Salad

Snack/Dessert - Peanut Butter Cupcake

Day 5

Breakfast – Buttered Omelet

Lunch - Cream of Asparagus Soup

Dinner - Cheese Broccoli Soup

Snack/Dessert - Peanut Butter Cupcake

Day 6

Breakfast - Breakfast Sausage

Lunch - Sautéed Cabbage with Corned Beef

Dinner – Keto-Style Chicken Salad

Snack/Dessert - Onion Garlic Yogurt Dip

Day 7

Breakfast - Keto Breakfast

Lunch - Chicken Pot Stickers

Dinner – Chicken and Bacon Roll

Snack/Dessert - Bran Cheesecake

Day 8

Breakfast - Egg and Cheese

Lunch - Fried Broccoli

Dinner - Onion Cheese Soup

Snack/Dessert - Keto Biscuits

Day 9

Breakfast - Breakfast Jerk Chicken

Lunch - Cabbage with Cheese

Dinner - Garlic Beef Stroganoff

Snack/Dessert - Banana Milk Muffins – eat in moderation

Day 10

Breakfast - Baked Ham and Cheese Omelet

Lunch - Cheesy Chicken Enchiladas

Dinner - Mushroom Chicken Recipe

Snack/Dessert - Fruit and Nuts Parfait

Day 11

Breakfast - Herbed Mushrooms and Eggs

Lunch - Cabbage with Cheese

Dinner - Cheesy Bake Veggies with Mushrooms

Snack/Dessert - Fruit and Nuts Parfait

Day 12

Breakfast - Basil Scrambled Eggs

Lunch - Cheesy Chicken Enchiladas

Dinner – Chicken and Vegetable Soup Recipe

Snack/Dessert - Spicy Trail Mix

Day 13

Breakfast - Basil Scrambled Eggs

Lunch - Creole-style Cabbage Rolls

Dinner - Cheesy Broccoli Soup

Snack/Dessert - Choco Brownies

Day 14

Breakfast - Baked Omelet with Cheese

Lunch - Grilled Chicken Salad

Dinner - Fried Spinach

Snack/Dessert - Refrigerator Fudge

Day 15

Breakfast - Cinnamon Pancakes

Lunch - Broccoli Quiche

Dinner - Spinach Tortellini Soup

Snack/Dessert - Zucchini Fries

Day 16

Breakfast - Ham and Egg Cups

Lunch - Japanese-Style Chicken Wings

Dinner - Sausage Cups with Sour Cream

Snack/Dessert - Microwave Tiramisu

Day 17

Breakfast - Avocado and Egg Salad

Lunch - Eggplant Parmigiana

Dinner - Chicken and Spinach Curry

Snack/Dessert - Red Velvet Cupcakes

Day 18

Breakfast – Spicy Omelet

Lunch - Chicken Salad Veronique

Dinner - Flank Steak (Slow Cooker Recipe)

Snack/Dessert - Vegan Nacho Cheese Dip

Day 19

Breakfast - Breakfast Sausage Casserole

Lunch – Asian-Style Chicken Wings

Dinner - Spinach Tomato Tortellini

Snack/Dessert - Nacho Hotdogs with Salsa and Guacamole

Day 20

Breakfast - Creamy Scrambled Egg

Lunch - Ground Beef in Mushroom Sauce

Dinner - Pot Roast with Vegetables

Snack/Dessert - Strawberry Cheesecake

Day 21

Breakfast - Avocado Lime Salad

Lunch - Glazed Meatloaves

Dinner - Tuna Salad with Pickles Recipe

Snack/Dessert - Peanut Butter Bites

Day 22

Breakfast - Avocado-Tomato Salad

Lunch - Broccoli with Garlic and Lemon

Dinner - Pan-Roasted Broccoli

Snack/Dessert - Colorful Cake

Day 23

Breakfast - Egg White Omelet

Lunch - Three-Cheese Eggplant

Dinner - Sesame Seared Tuna

Snack/Dessert - Layered Mocha Cake

Day 24

Breakfast - Asparagus and Prosciutto

Lunch - Pork Chop and Broccoli Bake

Dinner - Tuna Fry

Snack/Dessert - Tiramisu Cake

Day 25

Breakfast - Grilled Asparagus

Lunch - Spicy Buffalo Chicken Wings

Dinner - Buffalo Strips

Snack/Dessert - Coffee Cake

Day 26

Breakfast - Pepper Mushroom Eggs

Lunch - Roasted Broccoli

Dinner – Tomato Avocado and Olives Salad

Snack/Dessert - Carrot Cake

Day 27

Breakfast - Parmesan Buttered Asparagus

Lunch - Grilled Tuna

Dinner - Chicken Salad with Fruits and Nuts

Snack/Dessert - Blackberry Cake

Day 28

Breakfast - Romaine and Turkey Bacon Salad

Lunch - Pot Roast

Dinner - Ground Turkey with Hominy

Snack/Dessert - Carrot Fries

Day 29

Breakfast - Cucumber Salad

Lunch - Asian-Style Eggplant

Dinner - Lamb Tagine

Snack/Dessert - Cheesy Pear

Day 30

Breakfast - Broccoli Frittata

Lunch - Baked Sausage Balls

Dinner - Parmesan Chicken Salad

Snack/Dessert - Cinnamon and Peanut Butter Bites

Day 31

Breakfast - Cauliflower Hash

Lunch - Baked Pork Chops

Dinner - Tortellini Casserole

Snack/Dessert - Coconut Blueberry Bites

CONCLUSION

Cooking healthy and flavorsome meals that are low in carbohydrates is easy if you know how. This book contains a good number of popular dishes that are tweaked so that starch and sugar content remain relatively low, without losing the essence of the original recipe.

I hope this book was able to help you expand your culinary repertoire when it comes to low-carb meals and be able to cook on your own with the help of the recipes in this book. This diet may be a bit restrictive, but you can get the hang of it when you treat it as part of your lifestyle.

The next step is to try these dishes out for yourself, and discover (or rediscover) some of your favorites and make your own version. Hopefully, you can use these recipes as basic blueprint into making your own recipes.

CPSIA information can be obtained
at www.ICGtesting.com
Printed in the USA
LVHW021404020820
662080LV00006B/480

9 788395 666988